NO LONGER HYSTERIA

My Chronic Battle
with Endometriosis

TEYA FRIESEN

◆ FriesenPress

Suite 300 - 990 Fort St
Victoria, BC, V8V 3K2
Canada

www.friesenpress.com

ISBN
978-1-5255-5970-9 (Hardcover)
978-1-5255-5971-6 (Paperback)
978-1-5255-5972-3 (eBook)

1. HEALTH & FITNESS, WOMEN'S HEALTH

Distributed to the trade by The Ingram Book Company

LETTER FROM THE AUTHOR

There are a few things I would like people to know before reading this book:

1. This is my personal true story, not purposely intended to make people feel bad for me, but specifically for the purpose of sharing with friends and family, and anyone who will listen, the true struggle this disease is.

2. This book has been written by me with the help of my mom's memories of some events. Some people's names have been changed (this can be seen by the astrix * after the name). I received permission to use some names these shown without an asterix.

3. Thank you to all the people who have been, and who may start praying for me. Thank you to my family who has supported me, my parents who paid for my surgeries, my mom for fighting for me, and the friends who didn't leave when times got rough.

4. I choose to be vulnerable with all that has happened with me, not to gain pity but to help raise awareness of just how many parts of the body this complex disease affects.

5. Endometriosis can be found in a girl of any age. Don't just assume it's bad period cramps. I encourage you to seek help if your gut tells you there is a serious problem, and keep searching until you are heard...keep fighting for help.

6. This is a message to *anyone* dealing with something hard in their life... hold on to hope and *do not give up*! Fight for yourself to get the help you need and don't shy away from any opportunity to inspire someone else with your story.

7. Lastly, after writing my story and putting it on a timeline, I have experienced closure from much of what I went through. I've moved on with my life and have forgiven those unable to understand. My goal is to inspire people to live life regardless of what it brings. Thank you to all who helped, prayed for me, walked with me, and cared for me through my journey. I can never repay you!

Table of Contents

Chapter 1: Before Endo
(Age 0-12, 1997-2009)

My name is Teya Friesen, born March 25, 1997. I have lived in Winkler, Manitoba almost all my life (three years I lived in Steinbach while I went to college). As a kid I was a troublemaker with the brightest red hair. I was happy most of the time and was a big handful for my parents, but above all I loved life. I am the oldest and my brother, Reese, is two years younger than me. My family consisted of Reese and my parents until we got my dog Hershey.

Reese was always calm and gentle. He would admit when he broke something and cried so hard that he never got punished. I, on the other hand, would blame the thing I broke on Reese and he would take it because he was caring. Before Reese became a teenager, he was taught the difference between a pad, panty liner and tampon because of the many times I had to call to him from the bathroom and ask him to bring them up from my room. He would call up the stairs, "What color? Pink, blue or green," and I would pick a color and have a tampon or pad in seconds.

My dad, Loni Derksen was always caring and loving. We had tickle fights and I was always a daddy's girl. There was a time he was going to teach me to ride a bike but I told him I would teach myself. My mom and dad watched out the window as I fell to the ground, got all scraped up, but they never saw a tear from me. I had taught myself to ride my bike and my dad stood by proudly and watched that stubborn redhead do it herself!

My mom, Evelyn Derksen, was/is my biggest cheerleader in my life. No matter what happened between friends or me having a bad attitude she always cheered me on in the journey of life. She was the one I went too when I needed a shoulder to cry on when my friend Katie died, a relationship failed, or because I wasn't feeling good. My grandparents would also have a part in my journey as my Grandpa was praying for me and my Grandma had me down for many meals because I couldn't always make something for myself (thank you Grandma for all the meals).

I developed anxiety and stress as I had braces, glasses and red hair which were a great combination to be teased about. It was around junior high that my mom finally convinced dad that I needed a dog. She thought that he could probably help me with my stress levels. I was twelve at this time, and my life-long friend and supporter came to live with us in the form of a chiweenie (Chihuahua Dachshund mix). I named him Hershey. Little did I know, he would greatly help me with what lay ahead.

He was an abused one-year-old dog who was starved and every rib was visible. He was terrified of fly swatters, brooms, and feet because we assume he had been kicked and hit. If we moved our hand too fast he would shrink to the ground looking terrified. He wasn't house trained but he learned fast, as he found he was loved and safe. I was the first one who held him so maybe that is why he picked me as his favourite! To this day, if I go to the bathroom, he comes in with me, and if I go for a bike ride, he is in the basket on the front of my bike. And as he has gotten older, I bought a stroller for him as he couldn't walk very far anymore. He truly is a huge blessing in my life.

I didn't like people as a kid. I didn't want to be held or touched and I did *not* like hugs. I had few friends throughout school. My parents encouraged me to go to church youth groups, which I did, but I did not believe in God or want to make their faith my own. I didn't care if others hurt or were crying but I cared about animals and could easily tame wild animals such as chipmunks or squirrels to come eat from my hand and I could even pet them.

Also as a kid, I had lots and lots of energy. I had to keep going and doing something and two or three things at once was my normal. While playing with toys I needed the TV to be on, and also someone watching what I was doing or talking to me. I did lots and lots of running and playing, tickling and chasing.

I got ear infections regularly and this led to having tubes put in my ears (age four). My tonsils got infected at this age as well, and that was the second surgery I had. Once or twice I was in the hospital for dehydration being pumped full of IV fluid and in careful watch by doctors. Fevers were common, but less after my tonsils were removed and I seemed to have overall health under control.

The only thing I actually remember of that experience is Paw Print, my stuffed teddy bear that I still have today. He has a small paw print on his chest and he was given to me in the hospital just before the tonsils surgery. Right after surgery, I started getting nauseous and threw up all over my bear. I cried and the nurses told me they would wash him and dry him and bring him right back, which they did.

I had a severe sweating problem from grade 5-8ish which one of my friends was very disgusted by. I changed shirts many times throughout the day. We looked for ways to make it stop but couldn't. We now wonder if this was a sign that my hormones were going crazy and out of whack.

Chapter 2: Becoming a "Woman" (Age 12-13, 2009-2010)

This is the time I got my first period. I was at school (grade 7) wearing purple pants. My mom got a call from a teacher that they were sending me home because I got my period and it was pouring down my legs. My mom watched me walking home, across the school yard, crying all the way as my pants were getting soaked (we lived across from the school).

I didn't have pain or cramps with my period…it was just a gusher. My mom wondered how a first period could produce this flow but didn't think it was abnormal. Soon we realized that during the monthly periods I just *poured*. She took me to my family doctor, Dr. Brian* who said I should be put on birth control pills in order to regulate the periods for the first six months.

I started on Tri-Cyclin Low. The bleeding was a lot better on the pills and I stayed on them for six months. We hoped everything regulated and I went off of the medication, but it went back to the way it used to be. The doctor put me on them again, this time for a year hoping it would regulate my period.

I had one close friend Lauri, who asked questions about why I was on pills that 'pregnant' people use, and why I was using tampons when she hardly knew what that was. It sounded very scary to her, the concept of a tampon, but to me it was normal. It was the only way I wasn't soaking my pants throughout grade 7+8. Though she had many questions, she stuck by me. Through high school we would drift off, but still remained distant friends. Around our twenties we started up our friendship again and she again remained faithful to me through times of pain.

It was at the end of grade 8 that I started to complain about abdominal pain and severe cramps during my periods.

Chapter 3: Pain
(Grade 8, Age 13, 2010)

We went to Dr. Brian*, my regular GP many times about the intense pain that I was having during my periods. He gave me instructions such as relaxing exercises, and was asking if I was having stress at school. This is where the trips started, going to the ER with pain attacks. I was finding it hard to keep up with friends and missed about one day a week of school and more days over my period. Other doctors told me to take Advil, Midol or Max-Midol and sent me home.

We approached Dr. Brian* again who told mom and me, "some people have phantom pain and people just have to live with it forever."

I was hunched over and crying in pain and asked, "You mean you're not going to help me with this?"

He replied "Well, when there's nothing I can do, then there's nothing I can do."

My mom reassured me and told me, "Don't worry Teya we will figure this out. I'm not giving up." During this appointment he suggested having my mental health assessed by Eden (a mental health hospital in my city). My mom knew that I was not having mental issues; they were physical issues and that it wasn't *all in my head* (which was many doctors' "go to" saying at this point).

My mom knew I didn't need this assessment done but she got it done anyways. When coming out of the appointment the counsellor/assessment person told my mom, "She does not belong in Eden. She has no mental health issues other than depression which I can see why she has; this girl is really sick, she needs medical help not mental help. Go back to your doctor and tell him he needs to figure this out."

As soon as my mom was told this was a physical problem, she went straight to the clinic and had this doctor removed from my chart. She realized he didn't know how to help me, and it was time to see if someone else could figure out what was going on. She was determined to find someone who would help me.

It was important during this time to know that someone would still listen to me and help us figure this out, so we would go to the Urgent Care Center and ask the doctor for help. I was given a lot of advice, and medications to try for depression, muscle spasms and even for stomach migraines, all of which didn't work.

I was given Amitriptyline to try by Dr. Beth* in urgent care which did nothing. Nothing…was working, and no one seemed to know how to figure out what this was. It was very disheartening. Our happy life started to look bleak. I lay around for days in pain, and my parents' social life changed as they couldn't always make plans with friends, needing to stay nearby for me.

Chapter 4: It's All in Your Head (Grade 9, Age 14-15, 2011-2012)

On one of many visits to see a doctor, they suggested putting me on different birth control pills that might be better for me. I had been on a low dose birth control and it was time to change it as my periods had become very painful. Something stronger was needed. I started this new brand. At this time, I had a boyfriend who was trying to understand what I was going through.

After only a few days of taking it, I began to notice my shirts getting soaking wet in the front. I viewed myself in front of the bathroom mirror and didn't understand what was happening. Not only was my shirt wet, but my breasts appeared to be lactating. I went to my mom; feeling humiliated and asked her to come in the bathroom with me.

"Mom, there's something else wrong with me." I explained to her what was happening and showed her my shirt that had wet circle marks in the breast area.

"Teya, I have to ask you this to rule everything out. Are you possibly pregnant? You're lactating."

I was *shocked*. I knew I was always a troublemaker but I was never going to let more than one person have my body. This was the one main thing that I took from the Bible and felt it was a smart idea. "No mom...there's no chance. I'm still a virgin." With that, we tried to sew pieces of fabric into bras and became very creative taking a few pairs of extra shirts to high school, but I still felt totally embarrassed and paranoid. I would be going to the bathroom so often to wipe my front down and to change bras and shirts again.

After a few days of this, I refused to go to school because I was worried about soaking a shirt in class, so my mom started to investigate. What had changed? What was happening? She looked up the side effects on the computer to this new medication and read through all the side effects. There at the bottom of the page she read "some patients may lactate on this medication-however it's only a 1 percent chance." There it was....I was that 1%.

All options doctors suggested, weren't working so we decided to look elsewhere for help. We saw a Naturopath and tried Bioresonance therapy both of which showed there was inflammation in the body that affected many organs making them stressed, but that couldn't tell us what the underlying problem was.

Gym was hard. Not just because of the teacher or exercise/fitness but because I hurt. I was out of breath just making it to the top of the high school stairs and missed classes constantly. At one point, I stopped halfway up the stairs out of breath and a guy said to me, "You're so skinny you should be in better shape than that. You should try eating something." Little did he know that I had a ridiculous metabolism and ate *lots*, but I was always nauseous now and food was against me.

The thinness of my body was noticed by the doctors we would see regularly in our walk in clinic and also in our hospitals ER. On occasion we would hear something close to, "I know the problem here. You just need to eat. You're so thin. Do you know what anorexia is? It shrinks your stomach and then you're thin and always hungry. Just eat more and then the pain will go away."

I knew they meant well but when I had an appetite, I ate lots, and when the nausea and pain were too much, I couldn't eat very much. I was very aware that I had a healthy relationship with food. This wasn't the problem; the pain had increased as constipation was becoming a big problem.

Teachers tried to understand most of the time but sometimes did get frustrated with my lack of effort or focus and the many absences from class. I had one or two friends, but even keeping friends was hard. My best friend (pretty much my only friend) would stay. She would not only stay, but she would inspire me in so many ways.

Tamera never gave up or doubted my journey or if my pain was real. She was in grade 12, I was in grade 9, but that never stopped our friendship. She is legally blind, has a blind person walking stick that she claims is for whacking idiots (I think she was joking because I've never seen that happen) and has dark tinted glasses for her sensitive eyes. She has hearing aids and with them can hear perfectly fine.

You'll rarely see her without a smile. Even though I had a different life situation, she was inspiring me to keep going. I *never once* saw her sad, cry, or upset that she was blind. When we would go hang out together, I always drove and we linked arms and walked into the mall. She could see things if she holds them up very close to her face but soon she told me she was color blind on top of being legally blind.

"What? That's just super unfortunate, Tamera. Aren't you upset?" I asked her when she told me.

"No. Of course not. It's more funny than anything else."

She graduated and moved an hour and a half away for university. But on holidays and reading breaks she would come back home and we would instantly make plans. The usual was playing Just Dance on the Wii. Yes I could see the icons of what move to do next, but she had insane memory once she learned the moves even though she couldn't see the icons. Every single year, every single time I see her, I am thankful that she never left. Her mom once said to me, "It's not easy being friends with her. She's "different." But you two get along great. Thanks for sticking by her."

"*Hah*! I'm not the easiest either, we make plans and then I cancel often, or I'm too sick to make plans in the first place. She deserves a better friend than me."

She replied, "You've proved you are the best. You don't make fun of her, you help her, and you stayed." I couldn't understand why people would leave someone who needed help. How cold would someone's heart have to be to do that? That is when I realized Tamera and I were living the same life, she just didn't have pain and I wasn't blind. But we both needed someone who would stay, and encourage us. Since then we haven't been separated!

Due to missing many classes, the guidance counsellor was asked to collect my homework to send home with me on the days I did make it. She was very concerned and one day, when I made it to school, she asked me into her office. She was worried about what was going on and wanted to know if she could help.

I told her, "I just need someone to figure out my pain." She responded that many high school kids struggle with anxiety and this gives them pain in their stomach. She recommended breathing exercises for me to do and that I should come to her office on days I am at school and hurting and she would help "calm me down."

I had heard this diagnosis from so many people already, that I was furious. I told her that I knew that was not the problem and it was stupid for me to sit and breathe and think that could solve the amount of pain that even prescription painkillers couldn't help. Needless to say, I refused to see her again.

A few ultrasounds were given in order to try to find my problem, but nothing ever came up. One doctor suggested I see a kid's pediatrician for bowel issues as that can be very painful. The specialist said that I did have bowel issues (constipation) and I should start taking more laxatives and eating more fibre. Little did we know at that time, that this was not the underlying problem but a symptom of having endometriosis on the bowels.

Upon seeing one of the doctors at the ER, he figured I must be schizophrenic and had a problem imagining pain that wasn't there. He suggested we try a medication for this. Again we knew this wasn't the problem. We decided not to try these drugs, which had more side effects than we could see benefits. The pain was not all in my head as this once again implied. I couldn't understand why the doctor couldn't see how real my pain was. It was so excruciating and yet time after time, they were telling me it wasn't real.

On another ER visit, I was tested for gluten and lactose sensitivities because, "If your body can't handle milk or gluten this would really upset your tummy." Turned out I was fine there too. I was thankful for these tests as each test run was one more thing I didn't have.

On May 20th, my childhood friend, Katie, died after battling cancer her second time around. This was a shock to me to see how sick she was and how fast life was suddenly gone. The joy that she gave everyone around her would not be seen again in that way. I wondered if I had cancer, or if I had something worse.

Many thoughts went through my head, "At least Katie knew she had cancer. She knew what the problem was. I just want to know why I have pain." I looked up at the sky one specific time and screamed "JUST LET THE DOCTORS FIGURE OUT WHAT IS WRONG WITH ME! I DON'T CARE HOW SERIOUS IT IS JUST LET THEM FIGURE IT OUT."

The main reasons I said this were: 1. Doctors were refusing to help me because they didn't see a problem physically. 2. I wasn't able to make more friends, 3. I was starting to get suicidal, 4. I needed to know what was going on and, 5. I just wanted to be believed. I wanted to be able to show people and doctors a diagnosis so that I could possibly be fixed and I could start living like a normal teenager. I wanted my happy, pain free life back.

This was a very hard and dark time for me. I wanted to mourn for Katie and yet I didn't want people to think that all my problems were due to depression because I had lost a dear friend at such a young age. I didn't want the doctors to think once again it was all in my head as this was a traumatic event for me. I wanted this time to be about Katie and not about me, and yet my own pain and hopelessness was making that very hard to do.

Though Katie's death was hard on the community, family, friends and the school, it was not in vain. Her strength was a true inspiration to me and many others. She never complained and she kept fighting the whole time. You would never see her frown or upset. She knew she would die but she wanted to give others hope, so she created a charity called Katie Cares that donates money to other kids battling cancer.

No one knew the charity would get as big as it got. A portion of land across from the hospital near our city was donated by Morden Nurseries. In 2015 Katie's Cottage was built using the design Katie had made before she died. It's a place for people to stay when their loved ones are in the hospital. It's reasonably priced, and is just a short walk from the hospital. There was even a report that an elderly lady stayed in a room at the cottage as her husband was in the hospital. She said it was a beautiful place and that before bed every night she was able to look out her window and see her husband looking out the window of his hospital room, being able to wave at each other from afar.

This all happened over a few years but all along it gave me inspiration. I was transformed and noticed the things I could do, even though we didn't know what was wrong with me. Katie even had her own slogan before she died which I repeated to myself often. "See it...Believe it... Achieve it!"

Soon however, the days got darker for me; suicide was heavily on my mind but never attempted. Now looking back, I think the point where I felt totally helpless was one ER trip when Dr. Edwin* said "Hmm, the pain seems to be some woman issues. Just go get pregnant and that will fix everything." He was dead serious!

My mom and I sat there in shock. My brain began to run away with a million thoughts, 'is this what I have to do to get better? I don't want a child, I can't even care for myself most days.' I was simply terrified at this thought.

My mom finally asked, "Did you just tell a single fifteen-year-old to go and get pregnant??? You do know that this advice is a very terrible idea right?" He didn't see what the problem was, as he thought this would totally fix all my pain issues. We once again walked out of the ER feeling hopeless and deflated. Having a baby was not something to do to solve a pain problem and I was not going to have sex till I was married.

During another ER visit, my grandma took me to the ER as my mom couldn't make it and Dr. Edwin* was working in the ER again. He saw me and asked, "Are you rethinking the idea of getting pregnant, so you'll finally feel better?"

To which I replied, "No wedding ring equals no baby." He seemed very unimpressed by my lack of "trying to fix myself." I walked out hunched over from pain and anger and my grandma took me home as I cried the whole way.

Again I was going home without receiving help for pain because I could "fix" myself by getting pregnant. Grandma never asked what happened because she knew I was hurting enough. She just knew something bad happened, and was worried I may harm myself. So she waited upstairs in my house as I tried not to die in my bed till my mom got home. Technically she was babysitting me.

I believe eventually my mom did tell Grandma what happened. My mom only told me recently, that during that time, they had my whole family on watch for me. I was never left at home alone (which I thought was because I needed someone to bring me pills or help me to the bathroom, but really it was because they thought if they left me alone they would come home to a dead sister/ daughter.)

On the days I made it to school, I watched others getting boyfriends, laughing, having fun, having friends, going out and doing things and I looked at myself. A frail petite girl, who could hardly stand long enough to shower, had few to no friends, was such a hopeless cause, using breath everyday that I though others deserved more than I did. I felt people and doctors were all disgusted with me and cringed every time they saw me coming.

My parents worried for my mental health and suggested I see a counsellor to have someone to talk to about everything I had been through and was continuing to go through. Mom had heard good things about one in particular and I agreed grudgingly to give it a try. My dad sometimes even bribed me with McDonald's fries to go and see her.

At the beginning she was helpful, and it was nice for me to talk about all the appointments and ER visits I had, as well as the disappointments that came from them. But she was starting to talk about how the problem was really anxiety and how anxiety affects everyone differently.

When I tried to confront her and tell her I knew there was a different problem and I wasn't anxious, she reported to my mom that I had a problem with disassociation. She said the problem can only be fixed once I admit it. This made me more frustrated and eventually my parents couldn't convince me to go anymore.

Chapter 5: A Personal Lab Rat (Grade 10, Age 15-16, 2012-2013)

I was given a new doctor at the clinic. Dr. Chrissy* was a very caring lady who was shocked to see how thick my file was for someone of my age. She tried her best to help me by switching birth control and she wanted me to try a herbal route to see if the pain would improve.

I was getting headaches from blood loss now and pain attacks so bad I couldn't get out of bed. For sure on period week, I wasn't at school or out of bed the entire week. But I wasn't in school much anyways and didn't have many friends, or people noticing that I wasn't even there. I felt like I didn't exist to those in my grade anymore. Again we were determined to figure out what this was, and heard of a number of natural routes we could try.

We went to see a woman in Winnipeg who does NAET. This is a natural remedy to find and treat allergens in the body, which in turn could be causing my pain (but this didn't help for my pain problem). Locally we tried a physio-therapist, chiropractor, and a different counsellor. Each one noticed how tight my muscles were and tense my body was from pain but couldn't figure out where the pain was coming from. A few ideas were thrown around like it was my Vagus nerve out of place or too much stress in my life, but each idea didn't seem to fit what was happening.

The counsellor once again came to the conclusion that I was a teenager with anxiety. He started bribing me to go to school and push through the whole day of classes to learn to work through my anxiety. When I reported to him that I had done that I would receive a new stuffed giraffe for my collection at home. He was super excited that he was helping me; however, I still knew I had severe pain and wasn't getting better. It was *not* anxiety! I eventually refused to go see him anymore either.

I feel it is very necessary to take a second to praise my Foods Teacher, Ms. Grace Gibbs. She doesn't work at the school anymore, but she was a huge support to me as she let me do all the food assignments from home. I have recently contacted her while writing this book to tell her how much I appreciated her patience, caring heart, and grace. Her name has always really suited her!

It was in this class that two incidents happen. Incident #1: I was having a heat flash from all the meds I was on and walked into class with my hoodie off, wearing a tank top underneath like many other girls in the school/class did. A boy sitting by the door spoke up as I entered saying, "Oh my God you look anorexic. Put your hoodie back on." This ruined my spirits for the rest of the day. This was one of the rare days I had made it to school. Ashamed by my body, I put my hoodie on, worked in the hot foods kitchen and sweat like crazy.

Incident #2: We would be placed into one of the six mini kitchens in the foods room. Each group consisted of four or five people who would work together to make the recipe given. Sometimes there would be an EA in the room helping out, and this particular day there was. If I had to guess her age, I would say she was around sixty. My group was placed in kitchen number one which was also the only wheelchair accessible kitchen. Everything was lower to the ground but high enough for someone in a wheelchair to reach. The main cupboards were lower and built to have a wheelchair slide underneath the counter so they could also wash the dishes. There was no one in that class with a wheelchair that year, but it was still a perfectly fine kitchen to use, it just meant we did more bending down than the other kitchens.

I went and measured a few ingredients and brought them back to the group who worked on mixing them all correctly and preheating the oven etc. I usually designated myself to do the dishes for the rest of the time as the dirty measuring cups and spoons and dishes would come in, and doing them right aways meant less to do at the end of class when time was not always on our side. I bent over at a 90 degree angle to do the dishes because I was experiencing a lot of pain. Crunching in a ball or bending over hunchback were ways to help lessen it. It was normal for my group to see me doing this since the sink was lower anyways, and I always did the dishes hunchbacked.

This EA came over to my group and watched for a few seconds. She then walked over to me and said, "Why aren't you helping the group? The most important thing right now is not the dishes but making the recipe."

I looked up at her and said, "I'm not feeling well and I would help best if I could just bend over here and do the dishes. I have problems with chronic pain."

She scoffed, which turned into a slight chuckle and she said, "You're fifteen. You can't complain about pain until you're my age. Just stand up straight and help your group." I had heard this belittling before, but from an adult who was supposed to be a helper in the class I was shocked. But why should I start thinking now that someone would understand? It seemed nobody ever did.

So I stood up straight, walked over to my group, and asked, "Is there anything else you need me to help with?" The EA waited for their reply, but my group was so used to me helping them with the dishes they pushed a mixing bowl full of smaller dirty dishes into my hands and requested I wash those too so we had less to do at the end of class.

I have to admit, I was feeling like rubbing it in so I grinned a 'Hmm they didn't really need my help and I guess I was doing the right thing all along,' grin, which made me chuckle to myself, and actually, in its own way, made my pain feel a little bit better. I did enjoy proving her wrong in this case. Needless to say...she was not impressed!

On the other hand, one gym teacher was actually really sympathetic and was trying to understand. My mom talked to him about what was going on within the first or second day of gym class. One of his first rules for girls in gym was that he knew a period lasts one week so girls can't abuse that to get out of doing gym. But my mom explained I did have a constant period and that I was sick with something we were working on figuring out. Lorne Warkentine was very good about this. He said he still wanted me to be active but took time to see what I could do and what I couldn't. He told me not to overdo it when previous gym teachers told me to push myself to do fitness and exercise so my body would get healthier. I thank him for understanding.

I made many attempts to hang out/make friends with girls, but was let down almost every time. This was so hard to accept as it was hard to push myself through the pain to go out in the first place. I decided to no longer try, I just stuck with having my one girlfriend Tamera (who was still in University).

I was always hoping these other girls would be another true friend that I longed for, that they would understand my pain condition and would stay by my side no matter what. We would set a date and time to meet, usually at a restaurant or coffee shop, and I would always be stood up. I had tried desperately to go, making great efforts in my painful condition, and they didn't even have the decency to text me they wouldn't make it. I was crushed every time.

I watched from outside the window of my life as I heard girls in the gym change rooms talking about their period and how they took an Advil and it was fine. I was sitting there feeling left out, having no one, and thinking how an Advil would *never* work for my situation.

But through Geography class, due to my total lack of interest or understanding, I made another friend. His name was Tobias. It started off that we happened to be sitting together and he was trying to be funny but really he was making it easy for me to insult him. Now, it's not the mean insulting, but the kind that makes him laugh and those around laugh and makes the person try to insult you back. More like quick-witted humour! This is what our friendship was based off of; how red I could make his face (and he enjoyed it).

We started to hang out and became good friends. I got to know his family and sometimes went to his house. He got to know my family and came to my house quite often as I didn't always feel good. He didn't ask what I was sick with but he understood that I was sick. He didn't know why I always went upstairs to heat up the heat bag but he just enjoyed my company. We had lunch together (as Tamera was in university) and became jokesters towards each other.

Sadly, I wasn't able to hang out with him as much as either of us wanted. We remained friends during high school, and he didn't leave me because of my pain. Tobi was just one of those rare friends who knew the definition of a friend. Reese joined in and watched movies with us or played games, and so did Tobi's younger brother. It felt like another true friendship.

It was this year I told Reese how much I hated Geography because it was "pointless to have to study the world when I will just be living in Winkler all my life."

He replied, "Teya how many continents are there?"

To which my reply, literally without thinking, because the answer was so obvious was, "China, United States and Canada." Let's just say I was in Geography class all over again because Reese would not let me, "live life this way!" And thus, the Tobi and Reese duo helped me pass Geography!!

I would soon make another friend who would prove to be trustworthy and stay by my side no matter what happened. There were many medication changes, and cancelling plans, but he was OK with all of this, his name is Pedro. He was a grade below me but, somehow we connected. We were totally different in almost every way, but we were both Christians who just wanted to find trustworthy friends. We would hang out once in a while and talk about school gossip or just watch a movie. He sometimes asked how my pain was, but he had never assumed I was faking. He was great at encouraging me to keep going and to not give up, and some days I would only have him to sit with at lunch but at least I wasn't completely alone. He and Tobi would help show me that I was not invisible to the school as that is how I felt. We too, would remain friends for as long as I would remember.

Needing another school credit, I unenthusiastically signed up for Family Studies as I had heard it was an easy credit. The class only had girls (as could be expected) and Lauri was in it too. We sat beside each other as we didn't really know the others very well, and made small talk to pass the awkward class and time because our friendship had drifted apart over the last few years.

At one point in class, we were told to make a pretend birthing plan, watch videos on pregnancy and the labour process, and finally we would be given one of those baby dolls that are supposedly an exact representation of what it's like to have a baby. It would wake you up at night, cry during the day, make gurgling noises etc. and it was our job to figure out what it needed. It would scream and we had to change it (it senses if you actually change it), or feed it (senses if the bottle is to its mouth), or rock it. If we were too rough with it, it would have that information stored and the teacher would add that to the overall mark for that project. If we didn't hold it enough, or give it enough love/attention, that would also be sensed and saved and added to our grade.

I was *not* thrilled about this assignment. I felt like I was about to cry. All the girls squealed and talked about what they would name their babies, and about how much fun this would be. I held back my tears as I excused myself to the washroom. There, I tried to pull myself together, but I didn't know how I could. I would have to have this baby for three days, and I would have to take care of it. The problem was that I was not even well enough to take care of myself! My mom was taking care of me! I would never be able to have a baby with whatever sickness or pain issues I had.

During the time of this assignment, just as predicted, I couldn't do it. The baby had to be with me all day. I had to take it to all my classes and risk it crying in the middle of class, I had to take it for the rest of my evening and have it in my room for night in case it cried or wanted attention. The stress of having to lug this big car seat thing to class and have possibly to deal with a screaming baby in class was not good for me. I ended up just calling my mom to pick me up from school on the first day of this assignment (which happened on any day that I did even make it to school) and she had to come pick me up as my pain was skyrocketing.

It ended up being mostly mom caring for "my baby." If I didn't get enough sleep I would also have more pain, so she had to get up at night to play with this fake baby so she could go back to sleep in silence. Needless to say, I learned from this class that I was not ready to have a baby anytime soon, because I would not be able to care for it with my pain issues. This information I kept to myself as others would not understand and because of the numerous times I was ready to go and bury Baby Tyrell in the snow bank behind my house.

After so much of this chronic pain, my lack of friends and doctors not finding a diagnosis (I felt they didn't really care)…I was finally ready to die. I couldn't handle life anymore. I felt I was just wasting space on this earth and causing my parents so much stress. There was no hope for me to ever lead a normal life and the life I had now...I didn't want anymore. I watched my parents throwing money to this specialist or this professional for any hope of what could be wrong. It made me feel even more useless that they were wasting so much on someone who probably wouldn't be alive much longer.

My family sensed my hopelessness and they were very afraid for my well being. My mom, dad and Reese could *definitely* no longer leave me alone. I would be dead if I did not have support. I thank God for their love and wisdom and that I am still here today. My mom told me, "Teya, your job is to get through each day of pain, my job is to fight for you, and get you the help you need. I *will* figure this thing out no matter what I have to do."

Over my high school life, I had a few boyfriends and it was shocking to me that they were so kind and supportive about my pain when girls couldn't care less. The girls usually said something like, "It's just cramps...we all get them." I'm not saying everyone in high school was mean but many kids weren't really nice to me or seemed to care. They didn't acknowledge me (possibly because they didn't know I existed or was from their school) but some knew something was wrong and turned the opposite way to avoid the unknown of what talking to me might bring.

I understand now that they just couldn't understand a disease as complicated as this. We as adults, and even doctors, have a hard time understanding and I was being forced to grow up faster than them because of my pain.

I kept going to the ER, still looking for help and to hopefully find out what this could possibly be. Dr. Adams* announced at one ER trip, "We will keep her overnight. I am certain that the issue is stomach ulcers. We will give you meds to take and you will stay in observation." Staying overnight had happened a few times before when they wanted to monitor me for a while longer. Though I was a high school student, I had a special backpack with a phone charger, headphones, Bible, and a blanket from home packed and ready for overnighters. This helped me to feel as if I wasn't alone and a part of home was with me as family couldn't always stay with me.

One male nurse, a tall Jamaican looking man with long dreads and a Jamaican accent took pity on this tiny hurting girl. He offered me a strawberry ice cream cup with the little wooden spoon and I was blessed greatly. Upon noticing how grateful I was, he snuck me another but ended up cutting me off after three. Sometimes I truly just needed to feel like a person worth something, and not like a lab rat. After spending the night I was sent home to continue using the meds for stomach ulcers. This did nothing to relieve my pain. Another dead end, and another thing to stroke off the list.

Sadly, self-harm happened during grade 10. It was an attempt for me to try to be in control of my own pain. It seemed I had no control over anything in my life and I wanted someone to notice, someone to care, and something that I could have control of. I felt like a walking corpse, and seeing the blood made me feel a bit more alive. I am not proud of this downfall, but I now see it as necessary in my journey and a great asset as I always wanted to be a counsellor.

I had decided in the midst of all the counsellors I had seen, that I hated counsellors. So I would study up and become a great counsellor learning how to support, listen and show hope to others. Something I had needed and wasn't getting from the counsellors I saw. Thankfully, after three times of self harm, I realized it was very addictive and stopped cutting. I realized that that was not a healthy way of dealing with what was going on. My family was terrified for me and couldn't understand why I was hurting myself.

My appetite was another situation that my mom had to deal with. For the longest time she just thought I was a *very* picky eater. But as time went on, everyone in my family noticed that wasn't true. On one rare occasion, I was invited to a friends house for supper and they were serving ground beef. Previous to this, this was a food I was never able to eat. I would throw it up on the spot. When I cautiously stated that this was something I wasn't able to swallow, they told me "we raised and killed this ourselves, you don't need to be disrespectful and snobby and not eat it. Just put it in your mouth, chew and swallow." Afraid that this ground beef could be the way I may possibly lose a friend, I ate, I threw up, and I was sick for the next week.

Sadly the list of foods I don't like is longer than the ones I do like. My mom was so sweet to me, she made the family one meal and me something else, as there was usually something in it I couldn't tolerate. I was not able to eat/ swallow: ground beef, some pork, celery, cucumbers, tomatoes, Mexican or Chinese food, burgers, salad of any kind, carrots, or even chocolate. These things are still things I cannot eat, but I have been able to tolerate carrots now. Due to pain, I usually didn't do much so I didn't need to eat much. I was a tiny ten-year-old looking girl, who had one bowl of soup for lunch or who had a quarter of a box of Mac n' Cheese for supper. Breakfast, however, was a meal I loved and would have bowls and bowls of cereal. The thing I am thankful for is that I always enjoyed frozen peas and frozen corn as a snack or meal, and could eat this from bed.

By now I was doing most of life from bed. I taught myself how to drink any cup or bottle of water in bed, laying down flat, without making a mess. (I still use this as a bragging fact to my husband today, who needs to sit straight up in bed if he is going to have a sip of his water!)

Chapter 6: The Stoner Within Me (Grade 11, Age 16-17, 2013-2014)

I remember one clear moment, when I needed to make it to Math class in a few hours. It was early in the morning, 5am. I texted mom to take me to the hospital again for pain management and I was hoping to be helped enough to make it to class. Morphine was given and I was sent home. I arrived on time to math class which was SDL (Self-Directed Learning) making it a class of mixed grade 9-12's who wanted to do math at their own pace (or not at all for some) and with extra teachers help.

Heidi, a grade 12 girl who had always been concerned for me, looked across and watched me plop into my seat, drop my backpack to the floor and put my head on my math homework crying. My mind was so foggy, and I could hardly focus on math or anything else (honestly I was stoned out of my mind). I felt like a walking robot not able to think for myself, just doing the necessary things. Luckily this SDL math class was in a hut outside the school due to the overpopulation of students.

Heidi helped me up and we walked outside as everyone talked to each other about math questions and the teacher walked around helping those with their hands up. I fell onto the grass and cried pouring my heart out to her and telling her I needed to do my math, but I was stoned out of my mind. I cried, and she hugged me and listened. She had compassion and made me feel like finally someone cared. Of course, I knew my family cared but I needed to know there was more than just family who was there for me. Heidi helped me through that hard day and continued to check up on me once in a while before she graduated. To this day, we are still friends on social media and she has kept up with my health journey thus far. (Heidi, Thanks for your caring heart. You'll never know how much you helped me!)

A different day, yet again, rushed to the ER by my faithful mother; they shot me up with morphine (this was not uncommon). I was thin (about 100 pounds) and covered in many warm blankets to try to help the pain and stop me from shaking in the thin hospital gown. She assumed the dosage, inserted it in my IV, and then I waited. Soon I requested for my mom to get a pail, as I became incredibly nauseous. I started shaking, throwing up, and claiming to see things that weren't there. I'm not sure if I was overdosed or my body just didn't agree with the medication this day, but that experience made me think about why people would take drugs on purpose to feel this way. That was and is such a hard concept for me to grasp. I had to feel this way for pain and it was horrible. Why would someone want to feel this way on purpose and all the time?

This 'incident' impacted me for a very long time. The positive though, is that even though I was given and have taken a *lot* of hard narcotic medications for pain, I never once had the urge to abuse pills or take more than I should, or ever feel tempted to try doing street drugs. For this, I should be thanking God every day!

In April an abdominal sonogram was ordered and done by another ER doctor, this one for gallstones and gallbladder. The results came back...unremarkable with "no abnormality of the liver...no extra hepatic bile duct tract dilatation seen. The spleen, kidneys and visualized portions of the pancreas are unremarkable." Though this was hard to hear that yet again nothing was found, we were slowly making a longer list of things my pain was not!

Two days later my mom rushed me in again. This time I was kept overnight and given Maxalt (for nausea) and Toradol for the pain. By the end of my stay I was diagnosed with stomach migraines and prescribed Rabeprazole before I was discharged home. This was proven, also, not to work for my pain and was added to the list of things I was not sick with.

At the beginning of May, within a period of 72 hours, my mom took me to the ER three times. Each time we saw a different doctor. I honestly can't remember what the first doctor did for me, but it obviously didn't help as we went back when the next doctor would start his shift. My mom was quite emotional and asked this second doctor if he could please figure out what was wrong with me. My mom pleaded with tears running down her cheeks, "Look how thick her folder is, we are here *all* the time and nobody can figure out what's going on. If you can figure this out you will be a genius!"

He listened to my problems and read over parts of my file and said, "I'm writing you a prescription for Buscopan. She has spasms in her intestines." My mom replied, "No we have tried this medication before, and it's definitely not that." He wrote a different prescription, Dicyclomine, for the exact same problem and said, "Here she should take this. Then you'll come back and call me a genius." He left the room thinking he had cured me. We walked out once again feeling deflated and not listened to, knowing this was not the problem that I had.

My pain continued with a vengeance, so my mom waited till another doctor came on her shift. At this point my mom was very emotional and broke down crying to this doctor. Mom said, "Look how thick her file is. You're the third doctor we are seeing in a matter of hours. I really need your help. Can you please figure this out or order some tests to figure this out. We can't go on like this anymore. We're exhausted." I lay there curled in the fetal position crying my eyes out feeling totally hopeless.

The doctor then mentioned that she had seen us come in a lot, and there were a few tests she would like to see them do on me. She ordered a Pelvic MRI and an Abdominal MRI to be done in the next week but we wouldn't get the results until July. Then she asked a general surgeon who was up in the OR to come down and take a look at my abdomen. Once he was out of surgery and was able to come, he felt my stomach and suggested doing an exploratory laparoscopic surgery to see if anything would be found. We left the ER with hope, something we hadn't felt in a really long time.

The days came for the MRI's and sadly they couldn't be done on the same day. The nurse explained to me that I would need to have an IV line inserted into my arm so they could pump me with dye during the test. I warned them that I had terrible veins and they collapse often when inserting IV's. I assured them they wouldn't get it on the first try. The nurse replied, "I've done a lot of IV's… you'll be fine." I was not fine, the first time the vein rolled (which hurts) and I was left with tears streaming down my face while my mom was in the other room. They tried again on the other arm and the vein collapsed (again, very painful). I was crying and begging them not to do it again. I asked them to do the test without the dye, but the nurse had gotten a different nurse to come try, and I told them my mom needed to be here with me.

My mom held my hand and told me it was all going to be fine. This nurse succeeded and with tears I walked in my cold open back gown to the table, lay down, and went into the MRI's machine crying and begging God, "Why do I need to go through this? What have I done to deserve this? I just want to die… please have mercy on me and let me die."

Then I remembered in a few days I would need to do the other MRI test and I cried through the rest of the testing. Days later, I showed up with mom as my support, missing another day of school. This time they had a plan to try to save me pain. I was sent upstairs to the cancer ward to get the IV in as they are used to having terrible veins to work on. They got it on the first try and back down I went to have the test done.

May 30, 2014 would be my first major surgery (a laparoscopy). Over my few high school years I had missed days for a colonoscopy, gastroscopy, ultrasounds, blood work, urine samples, MRI's, CT Scans etc. These tests had been ordered here and there by ER doctors and they were frustrated seeing us coming back, day after day when nothing was showing up. I was so drained of energy that when I did share my last "adventure" with a friend from school, they never really had time to listen or made time to care. I was going to have an exploratory laparoscopy which was a time of hope from my mom and myself as we prayed that *anything* would show up. I cried out to God often and said, "I don't care if it's cancer or something worse, I just need to know what it is, and I just need the doctors to know that it's not 'all in my head'.

I was excused from all classes. I didn't know if teachers either didn't care that I would miss, or knew I had been going through a lot with my health, but either way I was thankful they allowed the time away.

My family took me to the hospital for my first 'big surgery'. Tears started to form as fear gripped me. Was I really this desperate that I needed this surgery? Was something going to show? Is this all for nothing? Will I die during surgery?

The questions never stopped. But some people from church had heard about this exploratory surgery and had put my name in the bulletin to pray for me, that an answer would be found. The youth pastor and a youth leader dropped by, just as I was going to be wheeled into the Operating Room. They took time to pray for me, taking my fear away and leaving me in tears that someone else was there to support me. I was still terrified, and wheeled away from my mom. Tears poured down her eyes and she still remembers how scared she was for me. Everyone was praying that something...*anything* would be found.

I woke up and searched for my mom through my grogginess. There she was waiting for me every minute and supporting me. She never left my room, waiting and praying. I asked her when my mind cleared up, "did he find something?" but so far she hadn't heard a word from anyone.

The next morning the surgeon walked in and informed me that they hadn't found anything, he did say however that I had fluid in the bottom of my pelvic cavity. My heart broke… tears stung my eyes and hope ran from my life. There was nothing, anybody could ever do for me; I would never have a life. No man would ever want to marry me, and my parents would be serving their daughter from bed for the next forty years. Feeling the pain from the places around my stomach where they had cut me open felt so pointless now. Why would I let myself get my hopes up just to have them crushed after all those tests and now this surgery?

It was here that I decided I would no longer have hope. I would tell myself nothing would ever fix me so my hopes wouldn't get crushed, and if something did fix me then I would not be expecting it and it would be that much more wonderful.

Now as my mom and I look back on this journey, a lot of fluid in the pelvic cavity is a sign that there is sickness present. We talk to women all over the world through Endo sites, and this is very common when Endo (inflammation) is present.

After this lap, we got the results for the MRI's and were told both of the scans showed nothing. We still couldn't figure out what was going on, so my mom had the idea of creating a medical binder to keep track of test results and medications. My mom asked for copies of all my previous tests. She decided to dissect each test and look up the medical words writing it up in "English." She noticed on the last test I had, being the Pelvic MRI that it said there was a thickening of my uterus lining and said, "endometriosis?" My mom was shocked to see that nobody had told us that they had an idea of what it could be. She was thrilled to finally have a possible diagnosis and answer, but I was not thrilled. I was not going to get my hopes up like all the other times.

Everything seems so sad. So I must add the one best memory that I can remember from this year. Tobi and I had the same History class. Again, we sat beside each other, this time by choice. This was a class that I hated just as much as Geography. "Why must we learn about the old times. Why can't we just live in the present. No one will ever use this knowledge in their life. It is totally pointless to someone who isn't going to work in a museum, or be a history teacher." Tobi found my misery enjoyable and would laugh, which made me laugh. He finally found a class where everything I said and the poor homework I did, he could catch up on insulting me (let's face it, he'll never catch up. But he did try!)

Now back to the happy memory! We had just learned about France and them branching off and making New France, and our assignment was to make a poster like they would have had back then encouraging the French to move to New France. The posters made us feel like grade 2, coloring a "Come to New France" or "Welcome to the Newness" (that was literally someone's slogan).

As I always did, I hammered it out as fast as I could. That was who I was. I would glance over at Tobi and see him using a ruler and being very careful. Yes, he is an artist, but this assignment to me was not important. I finished on the first day. We had three classes to make the poster either at home, at the beginning of the class or to finish the poster with the end fifteen minutes of class. We had the last few minutes to work on the posters.

Everyone talked to their friends while they worked, and some like me just sat there thinking. I began thinking about this week's doctor's appointments and how the last ones had gone, or thinking about my pain. I realized I needed to distract myself, and what better way than insulting my best friend sitting beside me.

I sat up in my seat and leaned over, "How's Mr. OCD doing?" He wasn't really, but it made him smile because he was particular with his artwork.

"Ha-ha" he said sarcastically. "This will be better than whatever you made. You were done in less than half an hour. I even took mine home and worked on it." He had just about coloured everything in and the teacher was coming over to us.

I studied his poster and let my famous smirk creep onto my face as the teacher arrived. "Doesn't that say 'Welcome to New Fance'?" He turned his head towards his paper so fast and read his poster. I laughed! I literally couldn't help it. He had put his words in bubble font and had totally forgot the 'r'.

The teacher noticed that I was right and saw he was greatly frustrated with himself. "Tobi, don't worry about it. Honestly, I won't dock any marks I know what your poster was trying to say. Just finish the rest up." Then she walked off. "You're horrible," he said trying to sound mad but couldn't.

I replied, "How can I be horrible? I just told you and the teacher, so she didn't think you needed to go back to grade 1 to learn how to spell." I couldn't help the smirk on my face or the insulting jokes that I said. He always shot back with a smile and used the rare times he could to insult me. It was a truly hilarious friendship, for anyone watching from the outside.

On yet another ER visit Dr. Scott* was confused by my case. My mom told him that I had had a Pelvic MRI done and he replied, "Yes I have seen it and it said there was nothing wrong." My mom pulled out her copy and said, "But what does this mean?" pointing to the possible endometriosis part to which he replied, "Oh that...that wouldn't cause this much pain." We knew that that was not accurate as my mom had already research and found that endometriosis is 1/10 most painful conditions. We were shocked to hear a doctor say it wouldn't be painful. Then we asked to be referred to a gynaecologist as we thought possibly this specialist would understand my pelvic pain and horrible periods.

In August, we went to see the paediatric gynaecologist in Winnipeg. She was a very kind doctor. Dr. Jamie* listened and said it was most likely Endo; however, she was surprised that the general surgeon had not found it with the exploratory surgery. She said we would treat this as Endo and laid out the options. Birth Control meds, Depovara shot, Visanne, IUD, or Lupron. She explained each one to us and the pros, cons and everything in between.

Over a few months we tried many different types of birth control meds. Most gave me severe depression as they wreaked havoc with my hormones. Each appointment I came back, having lost weight and feeling simply awful. I tried Visanne for one month during which I couldn't stop throwing up.

After still having all the pain, throwing up daily and not keeping liquids down my mom said enough. She called in and asked to be seen that day. We got an appointment for the next day as the doctor hadn't been in. The specialist took one look at me; grey faced with dark circles under my eyes, head hanging in a pail and having lost even more weight and said, "This pill is definitely not working." I weighed in at ninety eight pounds. Then she suggested we pull out the big guns!!

Dr. Jamie* suggested our next option would be Lupron. I shared this news of a new medication with my youth group and asked them to pray for me because I so badly wanted this to work and give me pain relief. Lupron is a drug that is administered through a large needle in the butt cheek. Each dose lasts one month or three months depending which dosage you get. It turns all your hormones off like a tap. You literally go into menopause.

At age sixteen, I was doing High School in menopause mode. I was having hot flashes so bad my mom wrote notes to many teachers explaining that if I needed to leave I should be allowed too. My pain did get a bit better but being in menopause is awful as well. I would be sweating severely, heat flashing *all* the time and started to get bad headaches.

Through this experience, I attempted to share it with a girl who I thought was loyal and I was mortified when I noticed other people started to figure this out without me telling them. I was bullied, being told, "Wow you look like you're ten, you are actually sixteen, and your body is acting like your fifty and shutting down!" I knew I was small and looked younger than I was, but the way the kids put it cut deep.

This medication was known to be so hard on the body that the maximum months recommended for use is six months. People that had used it before me had reported side effects such as: teeth falling out, hair loss, bone weakness and breaking, skin yellowing, intense brain fog and memory loss etc. But we didn't know this until after quitting the drug. Thankfully these things didn't happen to me although I did experience intense brain fog and still have memory issues. (This shot cost $500.00 each, and not a penny was covered by Medicare).

We continued going monthly to the clinic in Winnipeg to get this painful shot. Sitting in the waiting room was a hard thing to do, as everyone around me was either older or pregnant. I was totally out of place and felt so alone even though my cheerleader followed my journey. My heart desperately wanted kids in the future. I had just had my last month dosage and had now had six doses/six months of Lupron.

My parents, Evelyn and Loni were headed to Germany as my dad also dealt with chronic pain and needed a back and neck surgery consisting of removing and putting in four artificial discs. They were going to be gone two weeks but it ended up being three weeks due to complications.

Before leaving my mom talked to my younger brother about how he was responsible to take care of me. He shouldn't see friends too often and he should always check in on me in my bed and see if there was anything he could bring me. He should walk me to the bathroom or help me in whichever way I needed. My mom asked if grandma should move in to help, but my brother wanted to be alone, and I felt embarrassed to have a "babysitter"; however we promised to call grandma if needed. Then they left.

After about a week, I received all my pain back with a vengeance. The pain was worse than before (possibly from stress or from Lupron leaving my body). Reese contacted my grandma who had always been a faithful prayer warrior during my battles. She rushed over and we contacted Dr. Jamie* who decided we should come in, she would make time and we would figure out what to do. Almost throwing up and hunched over my grandma drove me to Winnipeg. I was so thankful that she was taking me but I also worried because my mom always came and she made the decisions on my behalf due to my foggy brain and my poor mental state.

Upon seeing me, the specialist recommended a three month dose (one needle) of Lupron ASAP. My grandma, only knowing that I needed help and not really knowing the facts of the medication said it was up to me to decide. I was in a severe pain attack and at that point would do anything to avoid what was happening in my body so I said yes. I did not know that six months was the max dose recommended, and the doctor didn't seem to be concerned with this fact either. My mom kept track of all those kind of things so I could focus on myself, on just living life one day...one hour at a time.

I was given the needle. It did nothing. It didn't work anymore for pain control and now it was in my system for three more months. Reese did the best he could caring for me, but grandma still had to take me to the hospital whenever he called. My parents tried to Skype every once in a while.

Once we got a hold of them, they asked how I was doing. I did not want to worry them as my dad was having a serious operation that could leave him paralyzed if something went wrong, so I lied and said I was doing OK and Reese was taking care of everything. "OK, if you're both doing fine that helps us to make this choice. We decided to stay in Germany another week because there are complications." My heart dropped. I looked down at my wrist and twirled the hospital band that I had kept on over the weeks to get in to the hospital a little quicker.

We said our goodbyes and wished farewell and clicked the off button on Skype. I broke down crying as soon as they couldn't see me and my brother hugged me. He was trying to be strong and to be around for me but it was too hard on him seeing me in such pain and knowing I wanted to die. Over the last few years, he had distanced himself from me as much as he could. I never really saw him because he never came into my bedroom and because I was usually in the hospital, at home sleeping, or I had food brought to my bed as I couldn't make it upstairs from the basement. That week was a terrible week. When Reese, Grandma and myself could finally go to pick my parents up from the airport, I could hardly wait.

As soon as I saw them, I ran and hugged my mom. Both of us had tears flowing down our faces and I had to tell her that I had an urgent trip to Winnipeg and I had gotten a three months dosage of Lupron which still was doing nothing to help.

"Normal" life slowly came back as my parents were home. But as my dad had just had a huge surgery, my mom had to split her attention two ways to try to help us both. I don't think anyone can grasp how strong she was during that time. She had two chronically sick people she was taking care of while trying to continue hairdressing from the salon we built onto our house. She also had a mother who had been diagnosed with Alzheimer's and was fading fast. Life was simply hard for her. She had no time for being sick or letting a cold or flu stop her. The other two in the family were much worse in health, and my brother was MIA most of the time as his heart hurt too badly to see his sister in pain.

Shortly after the last dose of Lupron, along with whatever depression meds or "other" meds the doctors had me on; I began to notice I had memory problems. One morning my mom came to get me up to see if I was feeling well enough to attempt school. She found me a little confused and my brain was very foggy. Throughout the next few days it all felt like a blur. She would mention things that had happened the day before and I was questioning her about this. Soon we realized my memory was getting worse and worse. I had trouble with school; after all you need to memorize a lot for tests and exams. I even felt different, like my emotions were gone. I had no feeling for anything or anyone. I even broke up with a caring boyfriend due to these new changes within me. I felt like a sad case. What was happening now?

I was sixteen-ish at this time and it was absolutely terrifying to wake up and not know your past, not know the things you did as a kid, not remember people. During this time of getting the Lupron shot and the pain being a little more under control, I attempted to be a normal teenager by getting a part time job at a Deli. I wanted so badly to do the same type of things my peers were doing. I also felt pressure as I was getting older and was making no money for my future.

Often after a shift I would come home and try to explain an entire conversation I had had with someone who seemed to know me better than I knew myself. My parents would listen patiently and try to figure out who I was talking about. "Teya, I know you don't remember but that woman who talked to you was your youth leader from a few years ago," or "that is your second cousin." I had no memories, I had no feelings or emotions. I was just totally lost.

One thing that I said to my mom when trying to explain this concept of pure emotionless was, "I feel like I could kill you right now and I wouldn't care and I wouldn't cry. I feel nothing and that is what's scary." Of course, my family knew I wouldn't hurt them...they were most worried I would hurt myself.

To this day, I still don't have many childhood memories. Mostly everything under grade 9 disappeared over night. I still run into people who I can't remember and it breaks my heart to know that this person and I somehow knew each other. Looking through picture albums of me as a kid at Disney World or me with an absolute favourite toy is the only way I know I did these things as a kid. This disease and these meds have taken those memories away from me. It stole years of my life in only a few months.

Side note,,,we now know that Lupron is not a safe drug. I would never recommend this medication to anyone. I know that not everyone gets all the side effects but hearing the stories of many who have used it, there are many with severe lasting side effects. It is just not worth the risk. At the time we were at our wits end and did whatever the doctors suggested since they all thought I was too young for surgery. Now I know better! Dr. Andrew Cook, a professional endometriosis excision specialist says this when it comes to if a girl is too young to have surgery.

> "The youngest girl that I have operated on was about eleven or twelve-years-old. In general, nobody likes to go through surgery, the decision to have surgery is really when the potential benefits outweigh the potential downside of surgery. The symptoms of endometriosis can vary significantly and their severity. What we are really talking about is quality of life. I do not believe that a young teenage girl should have to put up with more pain than her counterpart in their twenties to thirties just because she is younger. The process of deciding what treatment option is most appropriate for each individual varies and can be rather complex. Many factors are taken into account; the age of the patient is actually in my opinion a very minor consideration. The symptoms of endometriosis can vary significantly and their severity. What we are really talking about is quality of life. The main argument against doing surgery in young women is that the surgery is ineffective and she'll be going through surgery after surgery after surgery with the risk of forming scar tissue and other side effects of repeated surgeries. I disagree with this argument if a teenager is not responding to conservative therapy and appropriate surgical technique is used in the majority of patients she will have an increase in quality of life and she will not have recurrent problems in the future. Unfortunately, I still see women who have suffered for years and years in pain as well as women later in life that have suffered for numerous years and often the majority of their life.[1]"

A concerned cousin of my mom's had had some success with Sho-tai and recommended we go to Selkirk and see this natural professional. Sho-tai is a combination of different methods and techniques like reading the eyes, tongue, and physical body symptoms. It's a safe and natural way to perform physical, structural and nutritional analysis of the human body and the issues within it. It helps determine levels in each organ and area and recommends different herbal/ natural pills or juices to take to heal the body.

Appointments were made to go to Selkirk to have my body assessed. I would take all the natural herbs she recommended. We saw her every two or three months to recheck the things she had found wrong with my body the time before. She was shocked at how young and small I was and all the issues that kept coming up. She never once said the word "Endo" but she did say that she knew the problem was inflammation, hormonal issues, adrenal glands and liver. My PH levels were also way too high in my body. Throughout my grade 11 year and into grade 12, I took lots of herbal products three or four times a day. My constipation problems began to get worse.

Though Sho-tai proved to be some relief for me, the disease just needed to be removed for complete healing. Certain months I was given strict diet limitations which were hard for me to stick to but my mom *made* me. Sometimes it would be no cheese for the next two months, once it was natural sugars only for three months (*super hard to do*!) It was always different and not only did I suffer with these restrictions but my family all had to eat differently too. My brother never complained with the plain or gluten free crap that was on the table. We all ate the family meals and they did the restrictions with me to support me. I could have one meal a week as a "cheat" meal where I could have a small meal of one of my favourite foods. This would be the time I would plan for pizza with friends or chips with friends because most chips contain sugar.

This led to friends joking about my particular eating habits and how stupid it was to limit myself. I laughed too, but no one knew how horrible I felt. I loved food and could easily eat more than my growing brother. Some nights was just me crying in bed because of how much my stomach hurt from hunger pains, but there was so much I couldn't eat.

Chapter 7: Tijuana Mexico (Grade 12, Age 17-18, 2014-2015)

In grade 12, Dr. Jamie* thought the best idea for my health was to get an IUD (Intrauterine Device, basically meaning a flexible device inserted inside the uterus that's in the shape of a T). She thought it was another step in trying to control Endo. I would have to be put under general anaesthesia for the insertion of the IUD. This device would give off daily hormones, which should not allow me to have a period. This would hopefully help control my pain.

I was again allowed to miss school and we drove to Winnipeg in February. I was taken away from my mom to get undressed. I was small and cold in only a thin gown walking out looking for my mom but she was nowhere down the long hallway. It seemed like a horror movie because the lights were flickering down the hallway and doctors rushed around as if I was invisible. A nurse came up to me and brought me to a waiting room. I sat down with four other girls who all held their own box with the Mirena (IUD) in it (once again, something not covered by our health care). We all sat nervously looking at the floor, in thin short gowns. I held back tears. I was by far the youngest one there. This was yet another traumatic event and all I wanted was for my mom to hold my hand.

After that I don't remember anything. The next thing I do remember was being awake but my eyes still too heavy to open up. I could hear the nurses beside my bed talking about me. "Wow she's so small," one nurse said. "Probably because she's anorexic. Plus all these young girls just get IUD's put in so they can have all the sex they want and won't get pregnant." Comments like these went on. I don't feel the need to write them all in this book because they aren't important anymore but they were hurtful.

As I opened my eyes, I felt like I couldn't breathe well or talk. All I knew was that I needed my mom because I was worried. I hoarsely whispered that I needed my mom to the nurse pushing buttons on my IV monitor. "No you can't see your mom until we know you can go to the bathroom. You need to pee before we can bring in your mom."

"You don't understand," I replied, "You don't know what I've gone through. I need my mom, she will help me pee."

The nurse looked at me with her hands on her hips and leaned over. "Are you serious? You're going to graduate High School soon and you're crying because you need your mommy? All you had done was have an IUD put in. Girls younger than you are in here all the time and they don't cry." I just needed my mom.

"I am too dizzy I can't stand up." This nurse must not have understood that I was not one of the typical young girls having this procedure done as a birth-control method, so they could sleep around. I was in pain and just needed support. I was determined to pee so my mom could be called in but dizziness was stopping my goal from being achieved.

"You will be able to get up when you actually have to go," replied the nurse, snarkily. Too bad she didn't realize I was a stubborn and determined redhead. I grabbed my IV pole and drunkenly fell all over and finally got to the bathroom. I sat down and dribbled three drops; but who cares. I was going to say I had peed so I could see my mom. At least now I could say I did and technically I wouldn't be lying.

I went back stumbling to my bed and lay down feeling like I would totally throw up. The second nurse arrived to check on me and looked over the monitor again. "Do you have kids?" I asked tears streaming down my face as I lay there cold and shaking.

"Yeah I do. But they're brats." I looked away and replied, "At least you have kids. I'm having this done because they say I will never have kids. You should thank God everyday that you could have kids."

She looked at me upset and replied, "Lucky you."

I didn't stop crying all the way home from that appointment. The procedure made me feel violated, like I had been raped, and I was totally hurt by the comments of the nurses. My mom just had to sit there and feel helpless as I poured out my heart to her, my best friend. The IUD is said to last three years before needing to be replaced or taken out, but I lasted a week. It was supposed to not allow you to have a period but my body was totally rejecting it and I filled a maxi-pad every hour. I was faint, passing out, bleeding insanely and my uterus was cramping more than before. I could not get out of bed and going to the bathroom required help from family.

My mom called Dr. Jamie* to take the IUD out after only a few days. She told my mom that we needed to give it time to settle in. Her opinion was that I should keep it in for a month to let it start working and take effect properly. We said we would try and wait it out but my health was getting a lot worse and I was losing too much blood. After a week, my mom called again and told her we were coming in to have it removed.

We could see this had not been the right decision. I was in worse shape than before it had been placed, and this was really taking a toll on my mental health. Dr. Jamie* disagreed with our decision but said we could come in. After having it removed, I stopped bleeding the next day and improved slightly. This had been the last of the gynaecologist's suggestions. What would I do now? Was there anything else that could be attempted?

My mom, who was not willing to give up, kept researching to find a way that would allow me to be pain-free. My Auntie Brenda came to her one day with an article from the newspaper. It was a story about a girl from a neighbouring town, who had had surgery for her chronic abdominal pain. This looked interesting and sounded similar so my mom decided to contact her and see if this was anything that could possibly help me.

The three of us met at a local Tim Horton's and my mom did the talking for me; as I was in so much pain that I could hardly think for myself anymore. After my mom told her about all the doctors I had seen and explained what my pain was like she announced, "I totally know what that is! It sounds just like me before my surgery! It's called endometriosis! I no longer have it as I went to this amazing surgeon named Dr. California.* He is the best in the States."

My mom was thrilled to have someone who understood, but I on the other hand sat there in a sour mood. I had been "diagnosed" by so many other people and physicians. There were at least seventy other diagnosis before this woman and everyone thought themselves to be right. I couldn't have cared less what people decided to self diagnose me with. It was a mystery and I was living in my own horror movie.

Life was pointless. "She only has depression" some said.

Others bravely told me to my face that, "As a Christian you just need more faith and God would heal you." Little did they know that with so much time being in the hospitals in the last few years I had read through my entire Bible two times and had started reading it a third time. I had prayed and pleaded with God many times for healing, and my family had as well.

But, in the end, this woman's confidence and her journey ended up convincing my mom to look into whether endometriosis could be what took the beautiful joy and smiles, laughter and happiness, from her daughter those years ago. Could that MRI be correct when it said "endometriosis?"

My mom was excited hearing about this new doctor, Doctor California.* She immediately started collecting information on him. She went on his website and there was an area to ask questions of the doctor or ask for a phone call to discuss treatment with him. She left a short letter explaining what I was going through and asking if there was anything he could do for us. In a few days, we got a phone call from his office asking if we wanted to have a free consultation with the doctor over the phone. We excitedly set up a time.

In a few days the doctor called. He had a very calm voice on the other end of the line. He listened to my mom explain what I was going through and I explained the pain and exactly what it felt like. He said it sounded like endometriosis. However, he didn't want us to fly all the way out to see him if it was something else; so first he wanted me to do a breath test. He explained what was needed and how we would need to get a doctor in my home town to order this test for us.

He then forwarded our call to his receptionist. She was in charge of payment if we did decide to go to Dr. California* for surgery and it would be $40,000. We were a little concerned that he hadn't just told us to come, but that he wanted to be sure it was endo, and yet we were impressed too that he didn't want us to waste our money either. We considered the price, as that was a lot of money. Questions were flying through my mom's head, 'was this really Endo? Would this doctor really help Teya? Could we find another large sum of money as dad had just had a very expensive surgery as well?'

A few days later, my mom was talking to a customer in her hair salon about the chat we had had with Dr. California.* This woman mentioned a relative of hers from Alberta that also had Endo and had gone to Tijuana, Mexico to have an operation. We asked if we could have her phone number and my mom called her. She told us that she flew to Tijuana Mexico to see Dr. Mexico* for her pain. He had done an internal ultrasound, diagnosed her with endometriosis and then done a laparoscopic excision surgery to remove it. This gave my mom such encouragement that there could possibly be another surgery option.

My mom called down to Tijuana and explained my case. The doctor agreed that I would probably have endometriosis and looked over the scans we sent from previous testing in Canada. He called us to tell us he could help me and his price was $4,000. We thought that sounded way too cheap; what was the catch? Could we trust this doctor?

My mom called back to her new friend in Alberta and asked more questions about having surgery with this doctor. We learned that he was a very caring doctor who took the extra schooling in order to treat women with Endo because his wife had Endo and he wanted to help her. We heard how he worked in a top-of-the-line hospital and he had done amazing things for the lady in Alberta. We became excited, and decided to go see him. We felt we had found our answer.

We started raising money for the trip and possible surgery in Mexico by making and selling microwavable heat bags filled with rice. My heat bag had helped me so much and I wanted others girls dealing with period cramps, or anyone who injures themselves in sports to have a bag that can be microwaved or frozen as an ice pack to help their pain or injuries. During this time, my mom and I would sit and create. She would buy pretty fabrics, sew them together while I would cut the fabric, and fill the sections with rice, and then wrap them up with a string. It not only gave me something to do, but this project helped me feel like there were still things I could do.

During this time, a guy named Austin (he was a grade below me) who was a distant friend I had helped in the past, gave me $100 for my surgery. He wanted nothing in return. I broke down crying and was truly blessed by him. Another time, a man who lived beside my grandparents showed up at our door. His name is John. I had often walked across my grandparent's lawn to John's house and asked to play with their dog. I had done this for years before I became sick. Domino was their black Lab. He gave me many laughs and much joy.

John showed up and said he would like to buy ten heat bags (one bag was $10.00). I was blessed and let him pick out ten from all the patterns to choose from. He then handed me $200. I looked at him astonished and told him he had given me too much. He just looked at me with a smile and replied, "You just go and get the help you need. You deserve it." I started to cry. My mom came to see what was going on and when she heard the story, she cried as well. She hugged him with tears streaming down her face and thanked him many times. I cried long after he left. Not just for his kindness of money, but because he said, "you deserve it."

For so many years, I had told myself that I should just die because I was wasting my parents' money with all the expensive meds I was trying, and with all the trips to the ER. I was just wasting oxygen for those who were well and should live, and that I was worth nothing. I thought I would never *ever* get married because no man would want a wife who was sick, who can't work or even walk two blocks down the street. I couldn't even shower by myself, as many days I would get too weak and faint. For so long already, I saw myself as a burden, but maybe this surge of love and understanding would bring back the old me; the 'me' that everyone watched slowly fade as pain slowly worsened and took over.

I recently counted all the names we had kept track of when selling heat bags. We made and sold around 400 heat bags, many of which were to people who announced they were buying it for a daughter or a friend who had really bad cramps or periods. I was happy to hear that we could help other people who were hurting too. *Thank you* from the bottom of my heart for buying them!

My parents and I headed to Mexico. Reese would have come along but he wasn't able to miss drivers Ed class so he stayed home and took care of the house and Hershey. We took time in Mexico to walk some of the shorter streets and swim in the pool at our hotel before we would meet the surgeon/doctor. I was treated specially by my parents who bought me Pina Coladas (alcohol free) from our hotel restaurant. We walked a few streets in Tijuana, stopping at little gift shops to buy a pair of earrings or look at the unique things they were selling. All in all, we took pictures together, enjoyed tanning and the weather, while praying for help.

We met Dr. Mexico* in person on our second day there. I was put in a room alone with him, and questioned about all my medical history. I found this to be difficult as my mind was so foggy from constant pain, the medications I was on, and also I had been trying to block things out because I needed to live one day at a time. My mom was the one who remembered all the medication names and all the appointment dates.

Then he asked me, "I would like to do an internal ultrasound. Are you OK with that?" I was surprised to hear that he wanted to do this test. I told him they wouldn't do this test in Canada; it is considered necessary for a female to be sexually active before receiving an internal ultrasound. He replied, "That doesn't make any sense why they would not give you the test that could figure out all the problems?"

I agreed to the test, got the gown on, lay on the bed under a sheet and looked up at my parents who stood around me with a glimmer of hope in their eyes. I still clung to my new defense system of not having hope so my spirits wouldn't get crushed. I replied, "I've had many tests done. Bring on a new one…" The lights went off and the screen came on.

"Please put your legs in the stirrups." Oh my goodness, this was like the movies when the girls put their legs in stirrups and yell and give birth. It seemed so creepy to me.

Seeing as the lights were out, I put my feet into the cold metal stirrups. My dad stood by my head stroking my hair as he did years before till I would fall asleep. My mom stood by my side holding my hand. We watched the screens black, white and grey splotches show up. It was the scene from any movie when the woman sees her baby on the screen for the first time, except for me, there was no baby; there was a mysterious problem we were trying to hunt down.

The doctor was very good at keeping me calm and explaining what he was doing and what was next. "This may hurt, but I just inserted the device in and will be trying to find your uterus." 'Trying to find'…what did that mean? It was gone, had it just run away? The screen images moved and looked like nothing to any of us. Then the doctor spoke, "OK, so I am where your uterus should be, and there is nothing." A few seconds later, "I am on your right side and this is your ovary but there is no uterus."

I looked anxiously at my parents who looked down at me. These were the faces that gave me the most comfort as a man with a stick was going up places where the sun don't shine! "I am now going to check your left side." Everything inside my body started to flare up, angrily hating me for allowing this test and my face showed the pain. The doctor pointed to two images on the screen and said "here is your right ovary, it's in the right place, however your uterus has been pulled totally to the left side and has attached to the left ovary. Notice the pulsing of your uterus? It looks like it has a heartbeat."

I replied, "Yeah it is always cramping like that." My parents were surprised to see how bad my pain actually was and to have a visual of it.

"This is most definitely endo, and she will need surgery." At first we didn't move, too stunned at what we had just seen on the screen. We all hugged with relief and joy as there was some hope to be seen and we felt for the first time that we had a diagnosis.

The next two days were spent touring a little bit, but mostly I was sitting and stinking up the bathroom. I was given laxative pills that are to be inserted into the bowels as "clearing out" was needed before any big procedure. The bathroom was small but nice. I memorized it all from sitting in it so long. After the lax butt pills (not as fun as it sounds), I was required to take an enema. Yes, I did say enema. For those who don't know what this is, let me explain it in the least vulgar way. It's a bottle of liquid with a tube coming out the top that is inserted into the bowels and squeezed until all liquid is in your bowels. This makes you feel similar to the scene from Dumb and Dumber. If you don't know this movie or scene, it is easily found. Type in: YouTube "Dumb and Dumber Toilet Scene."

This was yet again, a whole new experience for me and I didn't know what to do. My dad made jokes to try to lighten the mood; such as, "remember, don't laugh or sneeze when you have the liquid in you. If you do, the wall will be a different color." This sounds embarrassing now that I recall this but in the moment I was thankful for his joking. I didn't want this to be a scary serious thing. He lightened the mood and this helped to put my mind...and bowels at ease a little.

This was my first major surgery (after the exploratory laparoscopy surgery) and I was scared. I asked my mom if she would come in the bathroom and help me with the enema. For me this was awkward but I also didn't know what to do, or want to go through this alone. I rolled on my side, back facing her on the floor and together we accomplished the task. She left as soon as the bottle was empty and I was left to squeeze 'them cheeks' for as long as I could and then quickly get on the toilet before the explosion. Frankly, lots of running back and forth, no food and little water, sweating, stinking and intense nausea kept me occupied up till the next day of surgery.

The next day I was signing Spanish papers (which felt like I was signing my life away). I had a poor translator and I wasn't sure what exactly I was signing for but I trusted the doctor and my parents. A few people at school had heard that I was headed to Mexico for surgery. Whenever I had entered the room they were in, they would joke that my organs would be harvested by the Black Market. Even though this scared me, it couldn't scare me more than the thought of being in this much pain forever.

When I woke up from my hour and a half surgery, the doctor explained everything he had done during the surgery. He had detached the uterus from the ovary, while saving the ovary. Both were in working order. He had removed with excision, (means cutting) the endo he found in the pelvis cavity. He also shaved away the inside of my uterus as some parts were thicker than others. It looked as if half the uterus "had grass growing on the inside and hadn't been mowed in a while."

He also found endo on my bowel so he had "carefully removed the sausage casing from the sausage without touching the actual sausage." (He had unique ways of describing his surgery techniques.) This explained a lot of the problems I had had with my bowels and constipation all throughout high school. I was so thankful he knew how to work in all these areas of my body! I was awake, and I was pain free!

I made it back in time for graduation. I walked into my high school feeling like a new me. The only pain I was experiencing now was from having an intense surgery, but this pain seemed minor. I no longer had 24/7 really bad period cramps. I was starting to feel like myself and I truly believed I wouldn't have pain again. I went to all the graduation rehearsals and started to act like my regular self, full of joking, laughter, smiles and energy! My family was surprised to see me bounce back so fast. I was not even taking the painkillers they gave me after surgery. The amount of pain I had from surgery was nothing compared to the pain I had before it.

This is where my mom noticed my strange behaviour. She would enter a room and see me lying curled up in a ball as if I had pain, and I was walking around with a microwaved heat bag. She asked me a few times, "What are you doing? Are you feeling OK?"

I replied, "Oh...yeah I am. I just feel like I am supposed to have my heating pad," or "Yes I am OK, I'm just not used to knowing what to do with my time if I don't have to be in bed." This was the hardest thing to try to teach myself. I had to work with my mind to know that I was well. I no longer had to take pain meds, I didn't need to have a rice bag in my purse or on my body at all times, and I no longer had to lie in bed doing nothing. I was well. I could go and run and jump, play and dance, walk and make friends. How could people even find enough things to fill their days with??? I did not know what things I was good at or enjoyed doing. I was used to being in bed so what did well people all do in their day?

My mind had been wired a certain way for many years, and this was a total 360 degree adjustment that I needed to make. Slowly, my family started to see me living the life of a healthy person; the person I used to be and had lost to endometriosis years before. I had a new counsellor who was very understanding and supportive and could teach me how to live again. He believed me and gave me many coping methods while challenging me to view my life in a healthier perspective.

Graduation day came fast. June 26, 2015 I was standing in a long line of graduates waiting to walk into the church with our caps and gowns. I heard fellow students around me complain about how hot it was outside, especially with the black gowns and caps on. No one really seemed to notice me, but my old friend Laurie and I stood beside each other waiting to graduate together even though we had drifted apart for most of high school.

I listened to the complaining and could not understand how they weren't excited that it was warm outside. They all had good health and they were moving on with life. The heat should be the least of *anyone's* problems. However, I kept quiet and smiled to myself the whole time bouncing up and down with excitement.

Just as we were about to be summoned to walk tactfully into the church, a boy behind me tapped my shoulder. I turned and noticed him. "Hey do you even go to school here or did you go to GVC Tech?" The high school I attended was GVC. But there was a smaller high school for those who needed smaller classes and more teachers help on the other side of town. They also taught some trade classes there, such as diesel mechanics and agriculture. This was the school he was referring too.

I smiled excited that someone was noticing me in life and said, "No. Don't you remember me? We had grade 10 Math together and I sat in front of you in grade 11 English. I think we even had grade 9 Phys Ed together too." (Somehow I had remembered him). He looked shocked and embarrassed. He turned away, and walked off to talk to one of his friends to avoid this awkward situation. My spirits were slightly ruined by this comment, but once walking in and seeing my proud family's smiles, I livened up again.

I sat up front and waited for my name to be called. I had fought so hard to graduate and now graduation was just minutes away. "Teya Derksen, graduating on Honour Roll." I looked at my parents with my mouth wide open in sheer surprise. *No way!* I had worked to keep up but I had no idea how I graduated with Honours. All I knew was that that meant I was 'kind of' smart! I walked down in front of the graduates beaming with excitement and took the Diploma. I smiled for a picture, and watched the proud faces of my parents and brother who sat in awe, just like me; I couldn't believe my ears.

"Teya has been chosen for a bursary of $250 from John J Janzen - Biblical Studies, one from Klassen's of Winkler $500, and finally, a Katie Cares Bursary for $1000." Everyone applauded and my mom even began to cry. They were so proud of me and I was excited and well! It was truly a blessing to have Katie's name said at graduation. She deserved to be there with the rest of us, but she wasn't. Hearing her name brought joy to my heart as I had tried so hard to 'walk like Katie' throughout my painful high school journey.

Shortly after graduation, I applied and was accepted to start College in September at Steinbach Bible College. Along with this acceptance email was a note, "Congratulations Teya Derksen, Steinbach Bible College has awarded you the Pastor's Scholarship..." I read out loud to my parents that this scholarship was worth $1000. I was thrilled that God was looking out for me. I hadn't been able to hold down a job throughout high school due to health so I was excited that this would help me pay for my schooling.

That summer after graduation, two articles were published about my surgery in Mexico in the local newspapers. On June 25, in The Winkler Morden Voice the article was titled, "Misdiagnosed: the pain of life with endometriosis." The next month, the Winkler Times published an article about my Mexico surgery titled, "Breaking free from the pain." I was thrilled that the newspapers cared about my situation. I was also excited that this would be a way to help other girls who were struggling with pain to reach out and get help. To have someone say "I believe you. It's real, it's not all in your head," was so important. The papers included pictures of my journey and me with my family, and my contact information for anyone wanting to learn more about this disease.

This paper was carried over 50 Km/31 Miles from my city and ended up in the lap of Michelle Sanders. She read the article and became emotional. Her daughter had been struggling with exactly what the article talked about in regards to what endometriosis pain feels like. Michelle contacted my mom. We all decided to meet at Tim Horton's.

This is where I met Stephanie Sanders for the first time. She was two years younger than me and expressed her feelings towards a disease that controlled her life. Her current high school experience sounded similar to the one I had just finished suffering through myself. We encouraged them to seek out Dr. Mexico* too, as he helped me so much. They too, tried a surgery with him but it was not aggressive enough and Steph's endo came back just as it would soon with me.

Dr. Mexico* recommended I go for Pelvic Floor Therapy in Winnipeg because of pelvic floor muscle issues due to years of pain. I didn't know what this was but I was willing to try. My mom scheduled an appointment and we had another one of our Winnipeg girls parties (they were never parties they were doctor's appointments). Pelvic floor, for those lucky people who don't know what it is, is a trained person massaging the muscles inside the vagina. It is not comfy and it is not fun. At the end of the appointment you are given exercises to do at home in order to help strengthen these muscles.

After this *very* awkward appointment I spent lots of time crying in the car to my mom about how I felt raped/violated. It was a woman who was working with me, and she was very nice but it was just too invasive for me. My mom understood but she asked me to try again as this is what the doctor had recommended and this would be good for me. Every other month we would go to Winnipeg and eventually it just became a regular non-awkward thing I did.

I learned to do the exercises she gave me (as well as tips on internal massage FYI was still painful to do) and it did help to strengthen my muscles. Then, when I felt them tighten, on my own I could relax them so I wouldn't have the start of cramps. That is how I made it through the summer up to college.

Chapter 8: College Year 1 "Embrace the Call" (Age 18-19, 2015-2016)

I began college in Steinbach, Manitoba pain free on September 3, 2015 feeling called to become a Counsellor. Every year the college has a new theme. This year, it was "Embrace the Call" based off the scripture Genesis 12:1-9. The daily chapel/ worship sessions were based around this theme as well. The idea was that no matter what God calls you to do, just embrace that calling and trust him and he will take care of the rest. Little did I know that this theme would impact a huge part of my life.

Two weeks later, just overnight, my pain reappeared with a vengeance. I was heartbroken. How could this be? We had found an endo specialist who had done excision surgery on me. This was not supposed to happen. What would I do now? Would I have to live like this forever?

My mom was also heartbroken with this news. I cried and told her "the homework is too much with being sick; there is no way I can do this." She encouraged me to try to finish the one year of school; telling me that it didn't matter what my marks were. It would just be good for me to live in a dorm and get to know other people. I felt like my dream to live a normal life had once again slipped out of my grasp, and my dream of being a counsellor would never happen. I easily slid back into my old pain management ways. I started carrying a rice bag and pain killers to classes and tried my best to act 'well', even when life was getting hard again.

I knew one girl at college who was from my hometown. Gabriela was the only person I really knew when I started there. She was the older sister to a friend back home. She helped me get to know where my classes were, learning what and how a syllabus works and let me cry when I felt overwhelmed. She knew I wasn't well and she did what she could to help me while I was away from home. Gabi lived in dorm with me and thirty-some other girls.

Having had a lot of trouble getting along with girls in the past, I found living in dorm, with others girls absolutely terrifying. I also felt the stress of living an hour and a half away from my family and not having my mom to help me do many things. There were double rooms or single rooms (which cost more money). I chose a double room mainly due to cost.

My family all came with me and helped me get settled in on move-in day and everyone stayed for the family wiener roast. I unpacked my room and was listening to the other girls laughing and talking in many rooms down the hallway when a girl with dark hair and glasses walked into my room. Jessica Lynn announced herself as my roommate. She said she was from Winnipeg and was very cheerful. She seemed to be doing way better with this move then I was.

Though we never really got to be very close, it was fully my fault due to my health. But the first week or two of school we really didn't know anyone else. We slept in the same room, so we went to the cafeteria together and sat together in the classes that we both shared. She talked about how she had a guinea pig at home and I shared about my cute little puppy at home and we exchanged pictures.

Within the first month of school, as we sat in our room writing papers for classes and digging into all out textbooks, I told her about my pain. I felt this was necessary as I now had a medications shelf in our room. Jessica believed me when I explained my pain, mostly because she didn't know my past, but also because of the evidence that started to show. The medications, the electric heating pad that was always in use on my bed, my need to nap often and some noticeable side effects from medications.

She soon realized I was not just a roommate. I was a roommate she would have to help out. Her kind heart was evident throughout our year as roommates. She was introverted (like me) and this led her to sometimes just staying on campus in the library writing her papers; partly because in our room I was *always* around but mostly because dorm was too crowded for her. Though she couldn't help me as much as I needed, she was making more of an effort than me to hang out with friends. Sometimes I felt guilty asking for cold water or a rice bag heated up in the girls dorm lounge but she didn't complain. When I missed a class that we were both in, she would always bring me the notes and help me understand what I had missed.

When she announced she had a boyfriend a few months after starting college (and it was a guy from the college) I was happy for her. I didn't realize at the time that this would mean she would be gone most of each day as his house was only a seven minute drive from the school. However, I discovered I really needed this to happen. It taught me that I could do more on my own than I thought. I still needed help and would sometimes text a different girl in dorm and they were always happy to help; actually happy.

The third year girls helped me out the most as they could see I was struggling and the third year students are always encouraged to help the "newbies" get the hang of college life. These girls really showed the face of Jesus in their actions. It brought about a new level of trust and love toward girls. I would like to personally say thank you to Kate, Gill, Ashley, Bre, Ha Min Ahn, Jessica (my care group leader, and from the Ignite team), Karlene, and anyone else I've missed.

There were also men on this campus. Some would commute in, just like some of the girls did and some lived in the boys dorm. Both dorms were on campus and could be seen from the school building.

On the first day of school I met my first friend, Vova. He was a seventeen-year-old, trying to learn English and was sent here to do schooling in Canada from the Ukraine. I learned that once you turn eighteen in Ukraine, they send you to the army and that isn't what his parents wanted for him. He walked me across the field from the school back to girl's dorm that first evening when the parents had all left and the students just hung out in the school getting to know each other. He was 6'4", had a unique accent, and his attempt at English made me laugh. He was always eager to let someone correct anything he said wrong. He caught on to English *very* quickly

Throughout the rest of our college experience he studied me to see when I was not feeling well, not smiling or in pain and he would make it his mission, as a friend, to make me laugh. He never failed to do that. He was such a good, caring, encouraging friend. Sometimes on an off day, at a class break, I would seek him out and start a random conversation. I did this just so that he could distract my mind from the pain and make me laugh in some way or another. Little did I know that he would marry Caitlyn from the Ignite Team (the team I would soon be on).

Everyone at school seemed so understanding and concerned, something I was not used to from High School. Even the Professors made it their job to know everyone's names, invite them down for meals or have private time after classes when they noticed someone who needed to talk.

After only two weeks of school, Gabi walked up to me in school and asked, "What are you doing now?"

I replied, "Nothing. Just going back to girl's dorm to be sick. Probably watch more Netflix or do homework."

"Great" she said super excited. "You have an audition for Ignite in ten minutes." "*What*??" It appeared that she had signed me up (to get me out of my comfort zone) for the college's singing team, Ignite.

Apparently, the best eight or nine people were selected to make up the singing team that would travel to churches, youth groups, and then at the end of the year, would travel for a week across Alberta. Not feeling good, and not at all liking public singing or speaking I freaked out. I went outside practiced 'Titanium' by Sia and walked into my audition.

At this time, I looked at the start times of all the people trying out. I noticed the name Jason Friesen on the list. My mom had happened to point him out to me on the very first day of school saying, "Oh Teya, look at him, isn't he handsome?"

I replied with, "Mom! You can't say that about college boys. And no I don't like him at all. He's not handsome." The truth was he *totally* was. But I knew I could not compete with 'well' girls; girls that didn't have health problems. Someone like him would never go for someone like me. So noticing his name on the list gave me a shiver as I tried to avoid him wherever I could.

I went in and stood before three music professors and the Ignite Director Pauline Loewen. They asked if I knew how to read music, "no", was my reply.

"Do you know how to sing on key?"

"Yes."

"Have you sung in public before?"

"Kind-of." I was not in much of a talking mood. I knew I was an average singer but I definitely didn't think I would make it on the team. I sang my part of the song did some scales and left.

A few days later, Gabi again approached me in school after a class embracing me with a hug. "Congratulations!" she announced.

"For what?" I replied. She dragged me to the bulletin board where Jason Friesen, Teya Derksen and a list of others I did not know, made it on the team. I phoned my mom and said, "Guess what? I made it on the team! But Jason did too. Ugh."

After her excitement of watching me step out of my comfort zone and participate in "life" a bit more she asked, "Who is Jason?"

"Don't you remember that guy you said was so handsome?"

"Oh my goodness, lucky you! Does he sing?" I sighed and told her he sings and plays guitar but it was no big deal.

Later I got to meet the Ignite team. The members were: Tyler Peterson, Jason Friesen, Derek Sawatzky, Sip (Joseph) Reimer, Stefan Kroeker (our sound guy), Caitlyn Shevchenko, Bre Mantyka, Jaclyn Goertzen, Jessica Klassen, myself, and the Director, Pauline. This would be the start of a beautiful friendship. Pauline had facilitated and led Ignite a few other times and was thrilled with this year's group.

At the end of the year, Pauline came to me and thanked me for being on the team. "I probably wrecked the team and made it more difficult with all my health problems and pain attacks" I said, as I hung my head in shame and embarrassment; remembering all the times the group had practiced without me or had to take care of me while I lay nauseous on a church pew during morning practice on the tour.

Pauline thought for a while and then said, "You are the one that held this team together. I have never had a team as united and strong as this one. They all had to work together and help you and each other. This has bonded the team in a deeper way. You inspired everyone, to push through anything because that's what you do!"

I cried when I was alone and thanked God many times for each of the people in Ignite. To this day, Pauline and I still connect. She has stood by my side through my journey. I finally had a strong friendship with not just one or two people, but nine other people!

Ignite is where I connected with Jason. He brought much joy to my whole family when we started hanging out. My parents were thrilled to see that someone was treating me so kind, caring, gentle and lovingly. We had all wondered if there would ever be a man who would want to take on the responsibility of caring for me through my health struggles, and he was my prince charming.

The thing that worried me most about possibly dating Jason, was that he had three other brothers. How was I going to explain what a normal girl's period is versus what I go through? How would he react to this information or would my history prove too much and make him run away? Would his family like me or would they want him to find someone who was healthy? And then there was the decision I had to make at the very beginning – should I tell him that my doctors think I may not be able to have children, or should I wait till he's married to me so he can't leave when he finds out?

Not wanting to waste my time or his, but also not wanting to let my heart become more invested; if this relationship might end anyways, I told him about my health, possible infertility, horrid periods etc. and waited. He hugged me and said he was sorry that I had gone through so much, and that those are all *not* reasons to leave someone. Wow! I was shocked. This was not the response I had gotten on previous occasions with people.

Meeting his family was also a worry of mine. Not all friends' parents under-stood my pain or accepted me, but his family would prove to be different! His three brothers were just thrilled that their brother had a girlfriend and it happened that I had graduated High School with one of his younger brothers. They welcomed me and overtime got to know my pain situation and *totally accepted me*!!! His family actually understood perfectly as his mom deals with polycystic ovary syndrome, which is also a painful uterus condition with the ovaries. All in all, it was a perfect family to be a part of and accepted into! We started dating December 18, 2015.

One time at school I needed Jason to drive me to the hospital just past midnight (school guidelines asked for dormitory students to be in dorm for night well before this.) He drove me and stayed for five hours, knowing he had classes the next day. He went back to school when he had to but at the beginning of each class when they requested prayer or praise items the whole class was praying for their fellow student in the hospital.

I had support around every corner, and caring faces that greeted me without judging me if I was not looking "put together." Jason appeared much like Reese. He has a very soft heart and cried when he had to take me to the hospital or had to see me in so much pain. He cried when he didn't know how to help me and he let me cry on his shoulder; often numerous times a week.

Brianne was also someone whom I bonded with. She had chronic pain all over her body. In her case, the doctors also couldn't figure out what was wrong with her. We never got close but we asked each other once in a while, in the bathroom while all the girls did their hair or brushed their teeth before class, "How are you feeling today?" We were not afraid to be honest with each other and we explained the new medications we were taking, how our doctor's appointments went, and how down and hopeless we both felt.

Though we had different pain, we *totally* understood each other and strived to be a "sick-buddy" to each other. Finally, after suffering a few years with her pain, she was diagnosed by the end of that year with junior arthritis in her body, and then re-diagnosed with tight pelvis muscle issues.

Of course, I could tell stories about everyone whom I went to school with because everyone was a blessing, but one more person deserves to be noted. Sheila was a forty-some- year -old mom, who was brave enough to join a college full of twenty-year-olds who were young and crazy. She had felt called for a long time to go into the counselling ministry and knew this was where God wanted her to start. You would never ever have been able to tell she was in her forties because she easily had enough energy to keep up. She had a great laugh, and there isn't a person in the world that could dislike her. To this day, we still make plans to get together.

Sheila became my "backup mama." I attached myself to her quickly and she took me under her wing. I started calling her Mama Sheila every time I saw her and by the end of first year the entire school called her Mama Sheila. "Just 'Sheila' would never be heard again," she laughed. To complete the year, she got her college hoodie and put 'Mama Sheila' on the sleeve.

Due to the fact that my pain was back, and pain attacks seemed to be coming more often again, I was often missing classes and trying to do make-up assignments. It felt just like High School all over again except the rules were stricter and you could only miss 1 ½ days of that class or it was marked Fail.

After the first few weeks of college, I dragged my drugged-up body into my Counselling Professor's office and cried. Professor Hali Reimer-Chaplin tried her best to understand my past history with this pain and what was happening now. She said that due to my absences in classes, I needed to talk to the Academic Dean before I missed too many classes. Otherwise, I was at risk of failing for non-attendance and would not be allowed to continue going to classes.

I went to him and began crying my eyes out again. I could hardly think, my mind was so drugged up. I felt slightly stoned but mostly I was in a brain-fog. I was having a hard time forming proper sentences and feeling like I was about to fall asleep every other minute. My professors worked together to come up with a deal - if I got someone from each class to be responsible to take my notes and explain them to me after every class, they would allow more absences. This took a lot of stress off me.

Many mornings I woke up with such bad pain but knew I would have to suffer through class because I didn't have any more absences left. Professor Hali had me in her office numerous times, trying to help me with what I was going through. She explained that if I chose to do another year at SBC, I would be required to do my Practicum for the Counselling program that next year or in my third year. I assured her I would not be back for a second year, I just wanted to finish this year and be done.

Once again, my mom was looking for ways to relieve my pain. She had heard of a chiropractor, in Winnipeg, who had helped others and decided we should give him a try. My mom picked me up in Steinbach and we went to Winnipeg. This chiropractor did Contact Reflex Analysis Testing and designed nutritional programs. He used alternative therapies and medicine to help people. I was tested and he could see all my hormones and adrenal glands were off but he didn't know why. We had a few visits with him and tried some of his herbal products. Still nothing improved. We didn't see him again after that.

As an early Christmas present, my mom presented me with a Tens Unit. Many endo girls from the endo sites she had looked at, said that the electric pulses given by the machine helped calm the muscle and helped a lot with the pain. I excitedly tried this too, hoping for some relief but it seemed that even on the low settings it was making my pain worse and my uterus was cramping even more because of the electric pulses.

I went home for Christmas holidays and was asked to help out at a company that sorted our town's recycling. It would be a short-term job for just over Christmas break. Though I still dealt with pain, I was determined to try to earn some money. Sorting recycling eight hours a day is mindless work. You sometimes forget what you're doing because it's so repetitive. For me, this was a distraction from my pain, as I was able to fill that time with talking to the other workers.

Kelsie was one of those workers who I already knew and who took time to understand the pain I had and cared. Later, we would even decide to go on double dates. I was thrilled that slowly even with my condition people were determined to still befriend me. This is also where I made a new friend - Cordell. Seeing as you're just standing there for eight hours sorting recycling it gives much time to laugh, joke, and talk to the person across from you. Together we were trying to collect all the paper from coming through. Cordell and I started talking and I said how I had a boyfriend Jason and he told me about his girlfriend Selena.

After a few days straight of working together and talking the whole time, I said, "Wow we get along great. You're hilarious and I could always use a good laugh. You know what we should do?" I asked excitedly. He looked at me and waited, "We should go on a double date and get to know each other outside of work! We would all be great friends!" I said with excitement.

We made a plan and I got to meet his girlfriend Selena, and he got to meet Jason. From then on, we would keep up with double dates. They quickly learned about my health issues and were very gracious. I even had to miss Selena's bachelorette party as a whole day in Winnipeg would have been too long for my health to handle. If I didn't feel good but was still up for hanging out we would go to their place and watch "stupid" movies together with chips for snacking and my heated rice bag. The types of movies we watched were, *Robinhood: Men in Tights, Monty Python and the Holy Grail, Hot Rod or Nacho*

Libre. They were always the ones to make all of us laugh together. We have remained friends to this day.

When I thanked Selena for understanding that we didn't stay too long at one time, and that I missed events she invited me too, she was so caring. "No worries! We always love spending time with you guys, even if you do have to leave early. You're health is by far the most important thing, and if that means we need to cut our visits short sometimes then that is totally fine by us. There's always going to be another time to get together!" I was shocked and cried for joy that God had blessed me with such understanding friends! At the end of holidays, I returned back to SBC with Jason and with my pain slowly getting worse.

By the beginning of 2016 by pain was as bad as before the Mexico surgery. In February, we made a request to see a gynaecologist in Winnipeg who was not a paediatrician. Dr. Danielson* was a doctor who, I noticed instantly, cared and understood. My first appointment with him was February 11. It was supposed to be forty-five minutes long and ended up being an hour and a half because he cared so much and time didn't matter to him; the person did. He looked over my entire folder of history and believed that Endo had returned. He explained that there are two types of birth controls. They are either estrogen or progesterone. Of course, they're not all the same amounts but they all fit along the spectrum. It's a matter of finding the right combination.

All the previous birth controls that I had tried hadn't worked properly because my body didn't need the extra estrogen but rather I needed the birth controls that fall on the progesterone side of the spectrum. This was so amazing to hear. We felt like birth control pills had always been pulled out of thin air, with no reason for trying the next one and no way to tell if the next would be good or bad for me.

Now, we knew that there was actually a way to find the right combination. He started me with progesterone pills but due to side effects we stopped. He then moved along the spectrum and started me on Evra, the Birth Control patch (mostly progesterone), hoping to steady the flow of hormones in my body to help control my periods. I was also given a suppository that I could insert in my vagina once per day, when I had pain. It was called Diazepam. He also said he would write a referral to the pain clinic to see if they would have drugs that could help me with the pain I was experiencing.

Lastly, he encouraged us that I should be seeing a psychologist; not because I was crazy, but because they can teach a person how to deal with the pain and have a more positive outlook on life and the future. He said, "Even if it helps 1 percent, it's 1 percent better than it was." I was told not to have my period again till the day I wanted to have children. Periods would only make my Endo pain worse so we were to avoid periods all together.

We walked out crying with joy and feeling like we had hit the jackpot. Someone who cared and someone who had shown us the options I now had and the options that I would have if these ones didn't work. He had not just a plan A and then "uh-oh I don't know how to help you anymore," but he had plan A-Z. He also noticed that depression was evident and put me on depression meds.

My mom drove me back to Steinbach where I met up with Jason and hugged him saying that I finally had hope that I could get a little better again and that someone honestly cared! He was thrilled to see me come back from an appointment and not be majorly depressed, upset or sad. It was what he had been praying for, for me. Even though we hadn't been dating long, we had always had to be open about all my "woman issues." He never thought it was awkward or weird he just accepted that that was what my life was based on at this time. Plus, my family had shown him that it was not weird at all for us.

Initially, he was very creeped out the first few times he came to my house from college. Listening to all the jokes my dad and brother made about the bathroom looking like a murder scene of blood, and about coloured tampons, was just a little over the top for Jason. He only had brothers at home so at first it was shocking to hear people talking like this.

But I sat down with him and explained that my life journey had been too serious, and my brother and I were forced to grow up very fast because I had woman issues thrust on me at a young age. Instead of all this period stuff being weird, we decided to joke and laugh about it so it wasn't always awkward. He understood after we talked about it, and since then wasn't so spooked by our openness. Plus, it was hard to be creeped out when my dad and brother's humour could make anyone laugh...especially when they didn't know that there is a line that can be crossed in joke making!

During the time that I was using the patch, I signed up to help at the college's faspa (that is a Sunday meal, consisting of buns, cheese, pickles and sandwich meats.) I would be serving tables and cleaning up the dishes, refilling the buns and so on. The people that attended were usually the donors who were generous in their donations to the college and anyone from the community that wanted to watch the program and donate.

While using the patch, I did experience hot flashes but not very often. While I was serving my assigned tables, I asked one man if I could take his plate. I leaned over with my formal T-shirt on and he noticed the patch barely sticking out on my shoulder. "Oh I see you have a patch. I know it's hard to quit smoking but it will be worth it." He smiled kindly.

I replied, "Oh no, that's not what it's for," I smiled politely, "I have health problems."

"Of course you do. You tell yourself what you need but I know a smokers patch when I see one." I was so incredibly embarrassed, upset and on the brink of tears. My parents and grandma had come out to support the school. They sat at a different table that I was not serving.

I went over and they could all see I was upset. "Please mom, I need to borrow your sweater. I will give it back."

"I thought you were hot?" my mom replied.

"I am but I need it." Noticing my desperation, she took off her dressy cardigan and gave it to me. I put it on and tried to continue serving my tables.

By the end of the evening, my family waited by the door for me. I gave my mom her sweater back. By then it was totally sweat through and I explained what had happened. Jason was there and heard and was shocked that someone had said that. They all comforted and consoled me.

The Evra patch was working quite well for the pain but I started getting a very sore, raw rash from it. We went back to Dr. Danielson* for another appointment. He suggested trying the Nuva Ring. Seeing that the current combination had worked well, he thought the ring would also be good for me. It is pretty much a plastic ring like a ponytail holder that is bendable/flexible and is inserted into the vagina. It gives off hormones for the month and can be taken out at any time to have a period. It is usually used for the month, taken out for a week to get a period and then a new one is inserted and so on.

I thought it sounded strange but I knew we were on the right track with the progesterone birth control meds because they had helped control my pain and finally didn't make me super depressed. This would be the miracle birth control that helped me. It helped for pain (not completely but decently). It helped me while my mom looked for a permanent fix to the problem; which is also what the doctor wanted for me.

I was taking Oxycotin for the pain and it also helped. Explaining this to my boyfriend of three months was not at all strange. Jason was always understanding and was just happy for any good news I could give him. I had previously explained in the least graphic way how difficult my periods were for me and some of my stories of hospital visits so he could better understood my "glamorous" previous and continuing lifestyle. He would even leave classes to heat up my microwave heat bag for me so I would be able to make it through class. Many girls were jealous of how caring and sweet he was. They all said how lucky I was to have such a sweet guy but they really didn't know just how sweet he was and how much he had to do for me each day.

It was at this time that my mom decided to once again call Dr. California* to see if he would be the answer we were looking for. She had been doing more research on him and realized that he was one of the best endometriosis specialists available. He was well recommended and I guess his price reflected his abilities. I hadn't taken the breath test he had initially asked for but we also now had proof that I had Endo.

A three-way phone consult was arranged: my mom on her phone from Winkler, Dr. California* in California and Jason and I in the student centre, on my cell phone. He interviewed us for a long time and Jason prayed that I would get help. He had gotten used to seeing me in pain but it didn't hurt him any less. Each time I didn't make it back to my dorm on my own he would walk or on occasion carry me back so I could get to my bed. He would also leave classes we had together to use the microwave in the canteen to heat up my rice bag hoping this would help me make it through class.

After talking for a long time with Dr. California*, he agreed that it sounded like my endometriosis had come back. He told us that there was an open surgery date at the beginning of April. He was ready and willing to take my case. This call took place at the beginning of March. The last week of school was exam week, which would end April 27. I broke down crying, hearing that I was sick again. I had known for a while that my Endo had returned, but hearing it from a specialist, who specializes in endometriosis cases and who had been a guest on "The Doctors" show, cut to the core.

Jason was supportive and hugged me and was very happy I would finally get the help I needed. After that call, I kept telling him he could still back-out of our relationship; he didn't have to date me. He could find someone who was healthy. He said that he was sticking by me. He said, "I don't want to love you, just for what you can do for me; I want to love you for what I can do for you."

The next week consisted of talking to all the professors about the situation. They agreed that I just needed to go get help. The arrangement they agreed to was that as soon as I finished all the assignments for their classes I could take the exams; almost three weeks early. I would then pack up my dorm room, move home, and go for surgery.

The next month was the hardest month I have ever worked. I hammered out ten page papers through pain killers and brain fog but I would *not* have gotten that all completed on time if Jason hadn't sacrificed much of his time to sit with me and help me put my thoughts clearly into the papers and help me find quotes from books to support my paper. He made sure I did the work but he helped however he could.

I passed all the classes I had taken. (List is at the end of this chapter if interested). Then, it was off to Los Gatos, California. This time we could make it a family trip with my parents and Reese. While we were away on this journey, my grandma was wonderful enough to dog-sit my dog, Hershey. After we arrived, we decided that seeing as we were in California, we may as well be tourists as much as my pain would allow. We messaged everyone back home that we were there safe and that it was warm and beautiful! Here is a quick layout of the trip.

April 9	Flew to Los Gatos, California, settled into our hotel and did some swimming in their outdoor pool!
April 10	Drove to San Francisco, went to Pier 39 where we saw sea lions, unique stores, Alcatraz across the ocean and drove over the Golden Gate Bridge
April 11	Consultation/ exam, and cleaning out
April 12	Surgery day

April 13 + 14	Recovery at the hotel, and sitting in the sun
April 15	Sightseeing at the Santa Cruz ocean/beach where I saw my first lighthouse, in person. We took a twenty-minute walk, ¾ mile through Henry Cowell Redwoods State Park (I made it through the whole thing but I did hurt afterwards). We saw Winchester Mystery House in San Jose. Following that was my appointment with Dr. California*
April 16	Flew home, Jason and Grandma picked us up at the airport!

My exam with Dr. California* consisted of nine vials of blood being taken so he could test for numerous things, including thyroid (which is a common condition that many Endo woman have.) I then had my consultation with him. He asked me many questions and looked over the last surgery images by Dr. Mexico.* "Notice your whole abdomen is this tanned color compared to the rest of your body?" he asked us pointing to my belly with my shirt up.

"Yes. Is that because of pain?" I asked. "No, that is because you have burned your skin from having your heating pad so hot." This was a shocking new discovery for us but to me it made sense. I often would not care how much the heating pad hurt my stomach, I just wanted the heat to reach my insides so they wouldn't cramp as much. He said he saw this all the time with Endo girls. Now I know better!

He made me show him exactly where my pain was located in my stomach and what it felt like. In a separate room, he did an external and internal ultrasound. He determined better where to spend time during the next day surgery by where I had pointed out my pain to be. He assured us that he would look *everywhere* but spend extra time where I said I had extra pain. He took a close look at my uterus during the internal ultrasound. He also showed us a new problem called adenomyosis. This evidenced itself when he pushed on certain areas of my uterus with the wand. When he pushed, there was a discoloration on the screen that went black, grey, and white quickly; thus showing him I also had adenomyosis.

This is a condition where the muscle that surrounds the inside of the uterus has endometriosis in it. These spots are very painful and can flare up at any time. During a woman's period week, they are often the most painful as blood gets caught and hardens in the muscle. Dr. California* explained I would still have pain from adenomyosis but that he could give me a Presacral Neurectomy. This was a procedure that would cut the nerve that runs from my brain to my uterus; in hopes of controlling the pain as this nerve was so used to firing off signals that I was in pain even if I wasn't.

He also suggested taking out my appendix. He did not want me to have any future issues with an appendix, and having it be misdiagnosed in Canada as if my Endo/Adeno was just flaring up. That could be very dangerous. We decided he knew best and told him to do everything he could to make me feel better.

My surgery with Dr. California* lasted an hour and a half. He reported to my parents as soon as the surgery was over that all had gone well. He said the last excision specialist, Dr. Mexico*, had done a great job but had not been aggressive enough in cutting out the tissue. He said that he had been much more aggressive. He had removed my appendix, which had endometriosis behind it, and my presacral neurectomy, was also done successfully. He had removed Endo from off the pelvic cavity, and checked all other organs for Endo. He confirmed that my ovaries still looked good and it should be possible for me to get pregnant though there was risk that with adenomyosis, I wouldn't be able to carry a child to term.

I woke up from surgery with lots of pain from the invasive cutting. I used my painkillers this time, but my pain only lasted for the next two days and on the third day I felt better. We decided to go look around and I even pushed myself to go on a short hike (though it was not a smart decision and I paid for it the next day with a lot more pain and stomach irritation).

At the follow up appointment, the doctor thought I was doing well. He showed me the video he had taken inside my body during the surgery and we watched his little tools cutting away little speckles that had caused me so much pain. He gave us a copy of the video and the images he had taken of the endo he had found on the pelvic cavity.

He told us the results of the blood work were good, however; he was a little concerned about my thyroid and suggested that I get future testing done. He was concerned that it could become a problem. He looked at my stitches to make sure they weren't infected and confirmed I was good enough to go home the next day. He made arrangements for me to see the nutritionist, who helped me understand which foods to avoid, which ones to eat more of and a list of herbal products that help endo women.

Fun fact: In order for Reese to be able to go on this trip, as he was still in High School, his Film Teacher told him to take as many pictures and videos as possible. On his return to school, he would be given the opportunity to make a presentation that would then be shown to the class. He was given a very nice school camera that he was able to take on the trip and he enjoyed taking over 3,000 pictures and videos.

He sorted through the best, and made a twenty-minute video presentation of the trip. He chose to post his video on YouTube to make it available to the public. To access this video (that contains Reese-type humour) and to see the places we toured, checkout the link located at the end of the chapter under bonus material. Warning: there are funny videos of me high on medication. These meds were given to me before my surgery. Also, my family (mostly my dad and brother) were just being who they are. They tried to see how many times they could make me cry or do weird things, seeing as I wasn't all "there."

We returned home during the college's exam week. I drove from my house the hour and a half distance in order to go and see all my SBC friends with only slight pain from the stitches in my stomach but that was nothing. I was excited to show them the new me; the 'me' that had little to no pain and who was enjoying laughing, running, jumping and playing.

I arrived at the campus and went up to the girl's dorm! Everyone was so thrilled and asked me so many questions. Jason walked over from guy's dorm to walk around the campus with me. It was a beautiful, sunny April day. Across from the soccer field, was a group of my college guy friends and I eagerly ran over to them and asked if I could play Frisbee with them. They too, were excited to see this new 'me' beaming with light and happiness, and acting like a healthy person. I only stayed for the day as I was done school and the students had to go back to studying for exams. So, I went home to be with my family.

I enjoyed my summer living as a healthy person. That summer I worked at a few jobs and visited Jason, who lived just fifteen minutes away from my house. He had lived so close to me all along but I only met him in College. Our relationship grew and slowly he saw a different, happier girl shining through; a girl with so much energy and love for the world!!

Bonus Material:

SBC Year 1 Courses: Semester 1 - Old Testament, Introduction to Counselling, Introduction to Psychology, Spiritual Formation, New Testament. Semester 2 - Biblical Interpretation, Life and Teachings of Jesus, Educational Psychology, Christian History, and a mandatory first years missions trip called MX 1 (mission exposure) where two groups were made including every first year and we spent time in inner Winnipeg.

Link to California video: https://youtu.be/oPFT9ww5ftA

Chapter 9: College Year 2 "Trust" (Age 19-20, 2016-2017)

Over the summer in July, Dr. Dennis* was assigned to be my next doctor. He was a young doctor with drive to figure things out. He was kind and did his best to help me as well as he could. He got me on the right depression meds, got me fast appointments, and he didn't give up on my case.

Once I started college again in September, I would request that my mom be signed onto my medical chart due to being in school an hour and a half away, and my doctor being in my hometown. This way she was able to: A) see results or appointment dates, B) come in the room with me as I was over eighteen therefore an adult myself, and C) talk to the doctor on my behalf when I was gone and relay that information to me. I would tell my mother which prescriptions I needed refilled, she would tell the doctor and the doctor was kind enough to send the new prescription to the pharmacy by my school. Having a doctor who cared and showed compassion was such a great experience.

Even though I said I was only doing one year at SBC to get the 1 Year Bible Certificate, God called me back. Going back to SBC in September was better than being there the first year. Of course, when you say to God, "I will never do that," he leads you right there. I was reunited with so many of my friends and could help out the first year students like the older girls had helped me. I was able to get the same room I was in the previous year.

I had heard that a girl from my hometown was going to be starting at the school; so, over the summer we arranged with the Dean of Woman that she would be my new roommate. Jessica, my previous year roommate, wasn't coming back.

Nikki became my roommate for my second year and together we walked into the first chapel for the new theme reveal. The banner was up for this grand new theme and it was the word I hated hearing the most. "Trust." When I had gotten so low with pain, all I could do was trust in something higher. For me that was clearly Jesus, as I had seen for myself the things He had done in my life and in so many around me, including things like miracles. Nikki was just thrilled it was her first year of college and that we were roommates. I was also glad Nikki was my roommate, but I was actually upset that this entire year, would be wrapped around the hardest thing for me to do, when previously I had had my pain attacks.

The scripture that went with the theme was Psalm 37:3-7. The Scripture was, "Trust in the Lord and do good; dwell in the land and enjoy safe pasture. Take delight in the Lord, and he will give you the desires of your heart. Commit your way to the Lord; trust in him and he will do this: He will make your righteous reward shine like the dawn, your vindication like the noonday sun. Be still before the Lord and wait patiently for him; do not fret when people succeed in their ways, when they carry out their wicked schemes."

Jason and I were excited to be just a six-minute walk away from each other here at school. It was so much better than the fifteen-minute drive back home. As soon as the boys moved into their dorm, the prank wars began. The first of many was one guy freezing another boys boxers to the front of a snowy windshield in winter. The pranks continued with glitter being put under the covers on one of the boy's blankets. They knew he would be coming in late and wouldn't turn on the lights, and would rush to class in the morning covered in glitter!

One spicy prank began with baking brownies only to have hidden hot sauce in them. Of course, these things brightened my days and helped keep my depression from getting worse. Although my medication really helped my depression still got the best of me every once in a while. After going through so many surgeries and traumatic events, even though I was well the depression still continued.

I reunited with my Counselling Professor and together we discussed what my practicum would look like. Professor Hali would be the one who finally found me the counsellor that I would open up to. She respected me and that would break down my wall with love. The practicum would allow me to experience counselling from the other side. The classes I had been taking, counselling focused, were teaching me how to be a counsellor. Now, I was required to be the counselee (starting January/ second semester).

This experience would help me to understand both sides to counselling. At first this did not thrill me one bit. My life was finally going great and no counsellor had ever really helped me yet. No one had proved to me, what a good, caring counsellor should be.

One day I drove home from school early on a weekend and had an appointment with Dr. Dennis.* My mother didn't come along for this appointment. We talked about my pain (from periods, and about me having adenomyosis) and he asked if I had ever tried this certain type of birth control that actually helped with pain as well. I said I couldn't remember, I would check with my mom and get back to him. My mother and I discussed this new med and decided to give it a try.

I was leaving for school once again so my mother suggested writing him a note with my decision in it so he could again send in the prescription for me. I wrote the note with my mom sitting beside me to help with the wording due to brain fog (a mix from Lupron and years of chronic pain). We decided it might be nice to add a Tim Horton's gift card, just to show a little appreciation for all he did. I wrote a note thanking him for caring about my situation and helping me get the medications I needed.

A week later, it was reading week so I was back home for the break. I was in the middle of having a bad pain attack from being on my period, so my mom took me to the clinic. We were going to ask why the new prescription had not been sent to the pharmacy yet and if this would help with this pain now.

Dr. Dennis* saw us right away but walked in looking at the floor. I was lying on the bed and my mom was sitting on a chair in the exam room. He set the Tim's card down on the desk and said, "first of all, I don't accept gifts." My mom made a joke about how she should have just brought him the actual cup of coffee instead so he could have quickly drank it. He didn't smile. He continued to look down at the floor. Then he said "There is a line between doctor and patient and that has been broken. I will no longer be your doctor." He continued looking at the floor. I was hurting and didn't say anything.

My mom spoke, "What? What do you mean?" Once again he replied with the same line. My mom asked, "Is it because we gave you a gift card?"

He replied, "I'm not sure if you're aware but your daughter wrote me a note."

"Yes I am aware, I helped her write it."

He looked sheepishly away and blushed. "I called the college of physicians and they advised me that I shouldn't have her as my patient." My mom and I just stared at each other. What was happening here? We were so confused.

"Do you think I have feelings for you?" I blurted out. Once again he blushed and repeated the same line. "So you're not going to help me and you won't be my doctor anymore?" I asked. I was referring to my current, ongoing cramping from my period. His ridiculous news was increasing my stress level which in turn increased my pain.

"That's right, I won't be your doctor but you," (he pointed at my mom) "I will continue to be your doctor."

My mom was furious, "Come on Teya, let's go." With that she took my hand, she turned and faced him saying "if you don't want to be her doctor, you are definitely not going to be mine." We marched out with tears on our faces and in total disbelief. He followed us out and said "oh I found her a doctor in the neighbouring town who will see her. A female doctor, let me get you the clinics number."

My mom turned around and said, "If I want to call her I have a phone book!"

We felt this was such a low blow. He had made himself, judge, jury and executioner and we had no say. We still don't know what was so upsetting to him, but we have heard comments that my case might simply have been too complicated or that it's just so upsetting to many that we went out of country for help. Either way, we did what we needed to do, and I'm thankful for that California trip.

That same month, my mom thought of a doctor who may be willing to take on my case. She personally asked this doctor if he would be willing to be my doctor. She told him the whole story about how nice Dr. Dennis* was and then how he took a note that we wrote together the wrong way and I was out of a doctor. He felt awful for what had happened and said he was more than happy to be my new doctor.

With that, I had a new doctor. I was nervous that I would once again do something wrong, but he was very encouraging. He was probably the best doctor that there could be. Dr. Maron* was so caring. His motto was, "You know your body better than I do. You know what you need," and he signed off on any painkillers I needed. He kept my Oxycotin filled so I could get some whenever I needed (around my periods) and he was OK with my mom talking on my behalf as I was usually away at school. He would keep my birth control prescriptions along with the others always filled so I wouldn't have problems.

He was truly a huge blessing for the next 16 months. Then he decided to move away to a different province, and we were left wondering if we would ever find someone as amazing as him again.

The famous, "all college retreat" was always at the beginning of October. It was a time when all the students would travel two hours to a Bible Camp and have a weekend off with *no homework allowed*. If you brought homework, you would be thrown in the lake (which was not warm!) It was a time for worship evenings, Bible studies, students getting to know students, playing icebreaker games and getting ready for another great year. Professors would hang out with us as well.

Friday we travelled and it was tiring. I still dealt with chronic fatigue from having pain for so many years. Jason and I sat together and the bus was noisy and full (about 120 people all together). When we got there we were assigned to our cabins (girls and boys separate of course) and I bonded with the few other girls in my cabin. Nikki was also in my cabin. This helped me to not be so nervous. I hadn't had much luck with making "girlfriends," in high school. Even in my first year of college it had been hard to try and put a lot of effort into making friends because of my returning endo pain.

I was a second year with few close friends but many acquaintances. The retreat started with unpacking, a supper in the dining hall, and icebreaker games. That wrapped up Friday. Saturday came and more games and worship lessons were laid out on our schedules. During the hours of free time, the students would surround a basketball court and play outdoor games. Although I was exhausted from all the activities, I still joined in and I was thrilled to still be feeling pain-free. Everyone stood around laughing and clapping, joking and making friends.

The evening came and it was a worship evening. The band played and everyone stood in the small building singing loudly with their hands up. We sang through songs with words like, "You give and take away," "One day I'll stand face to face with you," and the one that hit me most and got me bawling in joy was "Your tears will dry, your heart will mend, your scars will heal and you will dance again." Some songs got people crying and most words touched my heart as I was enjoying my newly found freedom from chronic pain.

We sat down on the floor in a circle for a prayer session. I was sitting beside Jason and Bre from last year's Ignite team. Soft guitar instrumental music was being played by one of the professors. The lights dimmed as the students and professors quietly sat in the circle praying for things that were on their heart.

But my heart hurt...no wait...I was starting to get pain. Right there, right then, I hurt. I hurt like before. It felt like a thousand knives stabbing me, my insides pulsing in pain, and everything cramping like it used to. My pain flared up, springing to life, worse than any small adeno flare from being on my period.

I grabbed my stomach and looked down with tears in my eyes. This can't be happening, this isn't happening. I'm just imagining it. But Bre and Jason who were used to seeing me holding my stomach noticed right away. They looked at each other and then at me. Tears flooded my eyes and flowed down my face and other students became aware of my situation.

Bre put her arms around me hugging me tightly but gently. "Are you OK?"

"My pain...my pain has come back. I can't do this. I need to get out." Bre and Kate and a few other third year girls helped me up and across the middle of the circle. I could hardly walk I hurt so badly, and everyone was watching. We got out the door and I could hear the whispers but that didn't matter right then. I collapsed on the porch outside the small building and cried in pain, laying there in the fetal position. The Dean of Woman and the third year girls tried to find my shoes in the massive pile and help me back to my cabin. Looking at the girl's faces, most of them were crying right along with me.

"This isn't happening," I said, to try to convince myself with words but it was. "Bre, is Jason OK?" I knew Jason was so soft hearted and this would crush him.

She looked through the window on the door and then again crouched beside me. "Yes there are a few other boys comforting him."

"Did I make him cry?" I asked.

"He's crying because he loves you and he's scared for you. But we are going to take care of you and keep him posted on how you're doing." We stumbled through the slight drizzle and over the slippery rocks, back to my cabin; which wasn't far but felt like it was on the other side of the world. The girls wept with me, and the Dean helped lead the way.

I collapsed into my bottom bunk mattress, curled up, and cried like a scared baby. "Jesus no. Please no. God don't let this happen!" Some girls couldn't handle seeing this and they left crying. The Dean asked if I had brought pills and I had. It was such a second nature thing for me that I hadn't even thought twice about not bringing them even though I was well. She got them out, and I told her that I was going to be stoned if I took them, was that OK? I asked because this was a Bible college. No drinking alcohol, no drugs etc were the Bible college rules.

The Dean said, "That doesn't apply right now. If you need the pills, then you need them. If you are stoned you can stay in bed tomorrow. Just come out when you can." I took two Oxycotin. She sent the girls away and talked to me as best as she could, but not understanding what I was feeling or what was going on. "Should I call your mom for you?" she asked.

"*No*! She would be devastated. You can't tell her. She paid for my two expensive surgeries and she desperately wanted me to be pain free."

"That is a lot of pressure you're putting on yourself. Don't think of that now, just think of getting well," she told me, stroking my hair and handing me tissues. That's right...again my new goal in life was to get well. Why was I so young and going through this? Going through this again! *Why*? She left soon after as I had requested to be alone. I then took one more Oxy because I was mad and in pain.

Jason had apparently met up with the Dean when she was on her way back from my cabin and asked her if he could see me with her supervision, but she said that there was one other sick girl sleeping in the room or else she would have let him come. He cried, but he had good supportive guy friends who hugged him and prayed over him the rest of the evening. When the third year girls and Dean returned to the worship/prayer session, they requested that everyone in the prayer circle pray for that second year girl, Teya. Everyone prayed, and some cried. I didn't know this was happening, I was just thinking of how I wanted to die.

Needless to say, it was the worst day of my life (or it's in the top five). Waking up that next morning I felt absolutely heartbroken. I couldn't tell my mom. She would only worry and she had worked so hard to get me pain-free. It would wreck her like it wrecked me. My head felt in the clouds, and my abdomen ached from having so much pain overnight even though I slept through it like I used to. This too, was a second nature thing that I had adapted to.

Nikki walked me to breakfast. Everyone who saw me either forced a weak smile or looked at the ground. Jason saw me as we got closer to the dining hall and ran over to hug me and ask how I was doing. People around us watched but no one knew how to respond. I remember thinking, 'Even though I put him through this much stress, he still isn't leaving.' What a unique feeling that was.

I began questioning everything once again. Starting with myself. Am I good enough to ever get married? Will Jason leave now? Why am I not meant to have healing? Will I live with my parents for the rest of my life, them always taking care of me instead of me eventually caring for them?

Then I moved on to questioning God. I was literally stuck at a place where God is what we studied and sang about, prayed about and thought about! And here God was probably looking down and laughing. He had me fooled again. He had me hoping and it was all just crushed. Why would a good God or a caring God shatter my world like this? Why do I believe in something that is supposed to protect me from Satan, but clearly just turned a blind eye to what had just happened? What did I ever do to deserve this? Why would God set me up for failure believing I could do a second year of schooling when it was hard to get through the first year?

I thought about my mom and wondered whether this would drive her to the edge where she would give up hope of her daughter ever getting well? Would she weep and cry for days at the news? Would she kick me out of the house and be done 'dealing' with me? Will she still fight for me or is all the fight left in her gone? Will my family still love me or will they love me less? Needless to say, I questioned everything even wondering if all my new college friends would leave, wondering if Jason would leave, and doubting that I could *ever* live a "normal life" again.

I had to tell my mom eventually, but I did wait until the next week to break the news. She was supportive and we cried together. She made it clear that as long as she lived she would be fighting for me to have good health. We now know that this was not endometriosis returning but this was the pain attacks from adenomyosis. It would no longer be constant everyday pain as it had been with endo, but flare-ups at random times. As adenomyosis gets worse, the uterus believes there is something that needs to be expelled and the pain I was experiencing was actual contractions. This type of random pain flares would be with me until the day my uterus would be removed.

Looking back now, it's funny to recognize how God always makes things play out for the better. My Thursday class, in my first semester, was Faith + Doubt and this was exactly where I was in life. I doubted if this Christian faith was what I wanted. It was difficult to sit in that class, as things were hitting me hard.

The professor had many comments that cut to my core. "It's not bad or wrong to doubt, because doubting shows you're trying to believe. It is those who are not doubting that we should be worried about. Doubt shows there is not a lack of complete unbelief." I felt better that I had been doubting and questioning God. That didn't make me a bad Christian. It proved that I was trying and by trying, making my faith stronger.

"Doubt does not stem from a lack of evidence, but from our sinful hearts. The solution for doubt is to see that God will do what he says he will do. We know through his word, and his loving disciplines that God does what he says. Doubt is not the opposite of faith. It is very valuable to us depending on what you do with it. This could be a positive way for us to build up faith; or a way to destroy us. Doubt can build us up, while unbelief is a choice to not want to believe."

"Being gracious on doubters can help them come from their suspended place and to a good place of belief. Doubt is the halfway stage between unbelief and faith. Doubt should lead us to further study and understanding, just like the story in Mark 9:24 where the doubter goes straight to Jesus. A more intimate relationship with Christ helps doubt and defines who we are. Resolving doubt will only happen as we search for answers in God. If our goal, in resolving doubt is deeper faith, we must always be driven to God." This was a mind-blowing concept for me!

I felt so much better about where I was in life and that doubting isn't a bad thing. For example: Job was an honest and humble doubter where he doubts God's character and presence while demonstrating faith and laying these doubts at the feet of God. His friends aren't humble at all and are "certain" about God and his character and speak words of judgment instead of encouragement because they spoke on behalf of God.

Job 42:7 shows God is upset at the friends because they didn't speak of God in the right ways but judged what God was thinking and why this was happening. Job humbles himself and says, "I do not know my God as well as I thought but God is not at fault, lacking, or the problem here." God rewards him for his honest humble doubting which leads Job to more faith and that is how I chose to go about my doubting and it did prove to build up my faith.

December 18th was fast approaching and Jason and I would be celebrating our one-year dating anniversary. I thought that he might propose on that day. On December 7th, my grandma (my mom's mom) died from Alzheimer's, just days away from Christmas holidays. This was hard news to receive but she hadn't been in her right mind for a few years already.

The funeral was to be on December 11th. Little did I know, that was the day Jason had planned to propose to me. He wanted it to be a surprise so he purposely didn't propose on the date I expected it. He talked to my mom and dad who had known of this plan for a while and told him not to change the date. "We need something special in the midst of the sadness and Grandma would still want you to."

So my dad took me out that day to do errands and I came home to a dimmed house with a tea light and a rose petal trail leading up the stairs and into the living room. There, under a large canopy, wearing a suit, holding a bunch of roses, was Jason. I said "Yes!!" and together we celebrated with a small photo-shoot in the living room. The engagement ring had been my Grandma's (my dad's mom). That Grandpa had died ten years previous, and as I had loved her rings, she wanted me to have them. It was, and still is, such a special thing to be able to wear my Grandma's rings.

It was a beautiful engagement day, but it was sad that my Grandma wouldn't be able to see my life. She hadn't seen or understood because of her Alzheimer's for the last two years. Before she got so sick, she couldn't remember words, but she had told my mom, "I don't care what happens to me as long as you take care of Teya and Loni and they can get well. If I could, I would take their pain and issues on myself." She was always very selfless and all she wanted was for me to be able to be well. At least one of us was now well. She could party in heaven with my other grandpa till her husband and family would also come someday.

When we returned to SBC after Christmas holidays, everyone congratulated us on the engagement. The days continued and Professor Hali was happy for me too. She explained that I could do my practicum during this next semester that just started or I could do it in my third year of schooling.

Seeing as I was doing better I would get it out of the way just in case my pain continued to slowly worsen like in the past. The classes I took were to help me get a career in counselling, but my practicum required me to go to counselling I agreed and my Professor selected a counsellor for me. After learning so much at counselling and finally having a good counselling experience through my practicum, I graduated second year of college along with Jason, passing all my classes!

Bonus Material:

SBC Year 2 Courses: Semester 1 - Marriage and Family, Romans, Faith and Doubt, Christian Theology, Christianity and Imagination and I began my Practicum. Semester 2 - Anabaptists History, Crisis Counselling, Conflict Resolution, English Literature and Composition, and MX2. (This mission's trip means splitting all second years into 7-10 groups usually around 5 people each to go up North to a community for a week. My group went to Grand Rapids to do ministry.

Chapter 10: Lessons Learned From Counselling (January - April 2017)

Quick introduction of this chapter: I took a journal to every counselling session that I went to. A requirement for my practicum was to be on the other side of being a Counsellor. Instead of learning all about counselling and how I could be a counsellor, I was tasked with taking ten, 50-minute sessions (one per week). This was to help me see what it is like to be the counselee and to better understand both sides of the counselling process.

Along with doing the sessions, I was to spend two hours each week, after each session, doing the homework she gave me or writing things that stuck out to me during the coming days. Mostly, I used point-form to write the things I learned from each session. This may not mean much to others who don't have chronic pain, but through this counselling, I was able to claim my old self again, and learn to have joy through my pain. (Please keep in mind that I did not have Endo pain at this point but I was expecting to be well and was dealing regularly with adenomyosis flare-ups. This pain is almost identical to experiencing birthing labour).

Session 1: January 19/2017 - Today I met my counsellor, Glenys. I think this counsellor might be one that I don't walk out on. She is not like the usual counsellors...just imagine a fifty year-old lady with bright pink hair, about 5'1, with a British accent! I'm not even kidding! She worked hard to understand who I am and what I had been through. She also tried to understand what I wanted to learn through this experience. She said something that really struck me, something that no one else had expressed before.

She said, "I'm sorry about what they've [doctors] done to you. You have all the right to be sad, depressed and feeling betrayed." I feel hopeful, that through expressing my story to someone who cares that I might find peace from some of my experiences. I thought it would be helpful to not just recall things from the past but to remember that I'm no longer living in the past.

I just thought of the quote from Kung Fu Panda: "Yesterday is history, tomorrow is a mystery; but today is a gift. That is why it is called the present."

Homework entry: This evening was a crying, fearful evening for me again. I doubted that I would ever be able to live life normally again. Food and fear, as a tag team, rule my life. After eating a cookie, I phoned Jason and talked to him about my fear. I was asking myself, what if that one cookie that brings back my Endo pain?(endo/inflammation feeds off sugar). I cried and asked if he would still marry me if I got sick again. I wondered what would happen after we got married? If I were to get sick again, would that make him upset?

He told me, "I started dating you before I knew you would have a surgery in California and be healed and that he was ready to marry the 'sick me' too." I appreciated what he had to say but I didn't want to be the "thrift shop teddy bear." This is the story I created to help others understand how I feel and view myself. Here is my story.

Thrift Shop Teddy Bear

"A little girl goes to a thrift store with her mom. She sees this teddy bear that is grey in color instead of white, with a missing eye and stuffing falling out of his side. She begs her mom for him and her mom buys it. Next week the girl goes shopping with her mom to Wal-Mart. They walk in and right there is a bin of big stuffed bears. They are brand new and clean with soft fur. They have both their eyes and aren't losing stuffing. The girl drops the thrift store bear realizing there is *way* better, and her mom buys her the new teddy bear." I feel I'm broken and not good enough. Why would someone ever pick me when there were healthy girls to pick from? I am worth twenty-five cents and they are worth $250. I'm worthless.

Session 2: January 26/2017 - I read Glenys my MCC bear story. She told me, "We're all MCC bears because of the fall of Eden." I am not Endo but I do have it. This makes me a fighter and that's my definition (not worthless) no matter what others say. I need to increase the volume on the good voices and shut out the bad ones. Who does Teya want to be? It's about who am I inside. I am the one who has lived my life. This makes me the expert on my story; thus only I get to define myself.

Homework: Listen to 'Blessings in Disguise', and repeat to myself that "I am made in the image of God."

Session 3: February 2/2017 - Who does Teya want to be? Glenys suggests: "A brave fighter!" On another note, I want to make friends but I don't know how because people don't always understand my sickness. Glenys replied, "You connect with people through experience, and sharing new experiences together. You will have to risk yourself because of your hurt from other girls in the past to connect; even though it means you may get hurt again. This is just another way you can be a brave fighter!"

I continued to learn during this session to allow myself to be vulnerable is how to make friends. In turn, I was hopeful that this could bring me healing. I told her I just wanted to hide and not try. At the same time, I did want to try to make girl friends. She assured me that we all like to hide; ever since Eden. Feeling depressed or sad isn't right or wrong, it just is.

Homework: YouTube video - 'Brene Brown Tedtalks on Vulnerability'.

Session 4: February 9/2017 - Do I take the risk at being vulnerable to live life as a healthy person and risk heartbreak when I realize it's hard or my Endo comes back again? Do I be vulnerable and believe I'm healthy or not get vulnerable/ get my hopes up to be disappointed? I feel anxious thinking about the idea of trying to live life as a healthy person. I need to notice when stress happens and where it is in my body (to be more self aware) and how does this make me behave?

<u>Homework:</u> MindShift App to help relax and becoming more self-aware/mindful.

<u>Session 5: February 14/2017</u> - I desperately long to live life normally. I'm grieving that I didn't have a normal life. I describe it as, "It was right there like a 3D movie. I grab for it and it's gone."

Glenys suggested I acknowledge my sadness by talking. I told her about how ridiculous some people act when they have a cold. They complain about a cold like they are dying. I said that it made me upset because I was dealing with so much more. Glenys helped me see that I needed to lay aside my judgments about other people's battles and mountains. Otherwise, my judgments would be like Jesus saying, "Teya your surgeries and endo are nothing compared to my crucifixion."

Rather, I need to join someone else and walk with them through their pain. I am trying to understand the saying, "thinking affects feelings and feelings affect thinking, so practice compassion so it affects your thoughts and feelings."

<u>Homework:</u> Observe the war that goes on inside my mind that makes others pain minimized and mine maximized. (I didn't go back for my next session until March because I did my second year missions trip up north).

<u>Session 6: March 8/2017 -</u> I realize how far I've come. I see my transformation from having two chronic pain diseases to one. I saw myself on MX (Mission Exposure) doing well, compared to how I would do in the cold if I also had Endo. The last day on MX, I had pushed too hard to do things in the cold so I had to go to the hospital nearby.

This pain attack was very bad, and I asked myself in the hospital, "Is this the time my Endo will come back, because I really hurt?" But I took my Bible and opened it up to the inside cover and saw the picture of Dr. California* and myself. Under that picture I had written, "Good health is a privilege, not a right." That's when I decided to live in the present, thanking God daily for health and not worrying about the future.

Glenys and I talked about Empathy vs. Sympathy: empathy draws on our own pain, allowing us to feel the depth of someone else's. Sympathy offers understanding and compassion for the pain of another. I need to allow my experiences to impact people; not to drive disconnect between us because I see their pain as less than mine. I am not able to judge what pain is or isn't and if I want to become a counsellor, I need to understand when I am judging and stop it in moments where it could lead to disconnection.

Homework: YouTube 'Brene Brown - Empathy video'.

Session 7: March 16/2017 - I am too scared to dream about having children or good health. The extent that we allow ourselves to feel sadness is as much joy as we can feel/find. When you cut off something because of the pain it causes or could cause you, you also cut off the possibility of the joy it could give. Just like I don't have hope in having children so I don't have to be disappointed.

Glenys said, "Even though your mom had a sick child, you brought her more joy than sadness." I am hurting my heart by living this way, not letting myself dream and limiting my emotions. There are pieces of me: like being a Jesus follower, a fighter, Jason's special friend etc, but if I feel the only piece I am is to be a parent and that doesn't work out, then the only way I defined myself is broken and I'm no one.

"None of us know if having children is possible until we try. How can you start daring greatly? You could do this by letting yourself dream. All you can be is who you are. If that's not good enough for others it's not your problem."

Homework: I will let myself dream by enjoying the moment and the idea of having kids.

Session 8: March 23/2017 - Do I want to embrace life as fully as I can? Well I've been called to live in a grey area. Black means no children and white means children but grey=???? I need to release my dreams and hopes that I push down to stop disappointment and my heart from hurting.

Glenys and I then started talking about Boundaries: We can't carry others' pain. We can have empathy for them though. We have a bigger God than "can not." "Let your dreams be a reality," said Walt Disney and I suppose it's better to hope too much then too little, because then what are you living for? And if one has no hope, they have no point in living.

Homework: Questions to answer: 'What does it look like and mean to live life fully'?

My answer: embrace opportunities and trials, live in today, not the future or the past, choose joy, be who I'm meant to be, not someone else, do the things I enjoy, follow my heart.

'What do you have to do to make it safe to dream again?

My answer: open up about my dreams, don't create defensive walls, allow my heart and mind freedom, let my mind be who it was meant to be and in doing all this, I will improve my quality of life.

Session 9: March 30/2017 (Jason came with) – Some things can't be fixed. Sometimes you just need someone to hug you. I have a deep longing to experience what our parents talk about (in regards to having children). A crisis means danger or opportunity, it depends how you choose to let it affect you. Children limit opportunity but provide others; they could be seen as a danger or an opportunity.

I now know I need to deal with emotions in a healthy way instead of shoving them down. I need to deal with my triggers (such as pregnant teens or abortions) in a healthy way, so I can dare greatly and embrace others joys (like them having children even if I don't know if I can).

Session 10: April 12/2017 - My journey so far (wrap up/ recap): Glenys has given me a safe place to learn change and I now have more space to have joy. This is because of my courage she helped me build. I have learned to choose *joy* in the midst of my pain. I choose to be happy that I have had this rough journey because without it I would not have been able to help so many people and learn empathy/compassion as deeply as I have. I have reclaimed who I am and I'm determined not to let the adenomyosis pain I am left with define who I am, how much I am worth, or steal my joy.

How do I reinforce what I have learned?

I do this by dwelling on who I am now, rereading these journal entries and feeling the joy of being set free to be myself. I believe I now have hope for the future instead of dread. I must continue to surrender myself to God and find joy.

First, to find joy you first need hope.

Secondly, you trust God.

Third, be aware that I can bring others hope through my completed story.

Fourth, the Holy Spirit is at work.

This was the cliff that God wanted me to jump off in order to soar on wings like an eagle. To see that he is at work, have faith and jump trusting his plan is better than my own for my life. Giving up control is the cost of surrendering, but you gain so much more than control was worth. Living in the grey area requires surrendering what control you think you have to God!!

Chapter Conclusion:

Through the counselling that I took for myself during my second year at college, I walked out a totally changed person. I had finally come to terms that I am still sick, and I chose to stop viewing my life as if I could be well. I just needed to accept that this is what it was going to be and stop seeing it as what it *could* be if I was well. I learned to be happy that I have had pain because through this I was able to meet Endo girls and have been able to empathize with others pain regardless of the kind of pain. It has built my faith up and made me a stronger person. I can finally say with confidence, I am not worthless I am a brave fighter!

Chapter 11: College Year 3
"Seek First"
(Age 20-21, May 2017- April 2018)

At the end of my second year of college, I practiced the things I learned about during my practicum and dared greatly, by trying to make a new friend, even though I remembered all the times girls hurt me. I started hanging out with a girl named Claudia who was also from my college. I explained to her that I didn't have any luck with making girlfriends and she said she totally understood. She became one of my closest friends and as it turns out, lives in a neighbouring town close to Winkler.

My mental health was great; I had a great mindset and my family was so impressed to see my progress despite random adeno pain attacks. I knew I needed money for my wedding and also for the next year of college as Jason and I both knew we had one year left.

I worked a crazy amount of hours at the recycling company as that job was distracting and usually helped me to forget about my Adeno pain (when I had it) until I crashed at home afterward from exhaustion and fatigue. I also did respite for a ninety-three-year-old man, at the request of his caring daughter (who would later become a good friend of mine, and the editor of this book!)

She paid well and together Jason and I worked hard and saved money as we prepared for our wedding and our last year of schooling. All this hard work and stress caused my adeno flares to increase which in turn caused severe fatigue. I continued to work hard and was just so thankful to be able to finally really work. I felt normal in that regard.

My mom helped a lot in preparing for the wedding! As the mother of a bride should do, I suppose! Jason said he didn't really care what I chose he just wanted me to run it by him before deciding, so he knew what was happening. We sat down one sunny summer day and talked about the wedding day. I told him, "I would like to do it Friday evening on August 11. Can we do that?"

He smiled and said, "Sure, whenever you want. Any reason why?" I told him that it was the day, seven years ago, that my grandpa died and I was wearing the rings he had bought my grandma. I wanted that sad day to become a happy day for grandma and for my family. Jason thought that was nice and that is the day we set. I ran this past my grandma to see if she was OK with this date, and she too was happy to turn a sad day into a happy memory as well. My grandpa's favourite colour (because he was colour-blind and could clearly see that colour) was yellow. So it became a theme colour for the wedding. Jason and I agreed on steel blue as the second colour.

Jason had three groomsmen: his college roommate from the past two years, Stefan; his childhood friend, Zach; and his oldest brother Andrew. I chose my last college roommate Nikki, Tamera who had remained my friend, even with both our busy schedules, and Deanna (Jason's oldest brother's wife). My mom and I picked out how the fake flower bouquets would look and her work friend (also her cousin), offered to make them.

When I got them, my mom and her friend surprised me by adding a special touch. Because my other grandma had died half a year ago, a pendant from her necklace was glued onto the boutique handle so when I held it I felt it and knew she was there too. All these small symbolic things were added, for the people I loved that couldn't be there with us.

Our families all helped out in different ways and on August 11, with the passage in Song of Songs 3:4, "I've found the one whom my heart loves," we were married.

In September we returned to college as a married couple! It was so exciting! On campus, in between boys dorm and girl's dorm were "the married people apartments." A small apartment building with six rooms usually for married couples, who were going to SBC. Our apartment was 350 square feet. The apartment included a bathroom, one bedroom (decent size), a kitchen and dining room/living room. Our kitchen table had to be placed against the wall, which meant it only fit two people sitting at it and was in the middle of the living room. Basically, we never lost anything because it was always a few feet away. Starting this new journey in our first place together was wonderful!

The theme verse for the year was Matthew 6:33, "Seek first..." Because we weren't in the dorms we were considered "commuters" and were part of a commuters care group which also included other married couples in it. The first care group was held at the home of a professor I had talked with in my first year about surgery and pain issues. She had told us beforehand to bring our swimsuits as they had a pool and a hot tub. I enjoyed my time in the hot tub as pain was still an issue for me. Just before we left, she pulled me aside and made sure I knew that anytime I had pain, I was always welcome to use her hot tub! What a blessing her kindness was!

In the first semester of school, I joined the Wisdom Literature class because I needed a certain credit. Again, I continued to make it to classes but some days were really bad with pain attacks from my adenomyosis. God always seemed to plop me in the exact classes that did *not* sound interesting to me but somehow I always needed to take them. God always knows best.

A lot of my life I had focused on 'why do bad things happen to good people?' Why was I sick, but the bully at school or a murderer in jail is totally well? Why did I have to go through this and why would God allow me to go through this? Little did I know that this class, the one I didn't want to be in, would help me understand all these questions that had been swirling in my head for so many years. This 'Wisdom Literature' course included Psalm, Proverbs, Ecclesiastes and Job.

Job had been a book that I had connected with but didn't really understand. I had always felt like I was living a life just like Job's. His story inspired me, some days, to continue to trust God and stay on the right path in life; giving up self harm, to give God back the control that I was trying to have over my life. I focused on Job and a few people focused on me. The students knew my history and listened intently when I had a comment to share in class. I didn't comment that much in classes, but I felt so connected to Job and I think I understood better than most of the others in that class, what he was going through.

Through this class, I learned that Satan can only cause the harm that God allows him too. God is still in total control (Job 1:12; 2:6). You can be the godliest person but still live in an environment of extreme pain, torment and suffering. Job's three 'friends' also resonated with me. Eliphaz, Bildad and Zophar reminded me of people in my life who had said things like, "If you want to be healed you have the ability to heal yourself. You just need to submit to God the area you are holding back." "If you had true faith of a mustard seed you would be healed." "Just have more faith and you will be healed."

All these things people have literally said to my face. Adults and elderly people alike, and sometimes it would be another person I went to youth with. Job's friends were the same way. Eliphaz saying, "just submit to God and good things will come to you (Job 22:21)."

Bildad, "No man is good so don't expect God to bless you (Job 9:2)."

And Zophar reasoning that Job's punishment was no less than can be reasonably expected and that God's punishments are based on your unconfessed sins (Job 11:13-16)."

The most shocking realizations for me from studying this book was that I can be angry at God, because he is *big* enough to take it! Job, throughout the story, took his problems, worries, anger and concerns to God. But his "friends" condemned Job and told him all the things he was doing wrong. Instead, they should have prayed for Job. Job declares that God is God (even when He seems not to be holy, wise, just and good). Talk to God instead of 'about God'!

This class, though very inspiring was a tough wake up call for many people including myself. But through it, I learned it is OK to be mad at God and that these emotions and feelings don't make you a bad Christian when you have times of doubt and anger towards Him.

In October I started to have more pain attacks than usual. One of these attacks led to a late night hospital trip with Jason. One weekend when Jason and I went home to stay with one of our parents for the weekend, I went to the clinic to see my family doctor, Dr. Maron.* He knew my chart thoroughly and all the painkillers I had tried. He suggested that I try Medical Marijuana to see whether that would help in the times I needed it.

Medical Marijuana is made up of two components. CBD which is the part that helps with pain and THC which is the part that makes you high (but for certain people it is the part that helps them with pain). Long story short, I took CBD only and it did help my pain a lot, but caused insomnia for the next two days straight. Sadly, it was not covered by our healthcare even if prescribed by a doctor.

During this time, my mom researched and found another way to use the Medical Marijuana that the doctor prescribed. Women on the Endo Facebook Groups talked about making suppositories to put right where the pain was located. It had helped a number of women, so we felt it was worth a try. My mom was given "the recipe" in one of the Endo groups and made the suppositories. My mom melted Cocoa Butter tablets in a saucepan added a few drops of the Marijuana oil and poured the mixture into a small mould, all this being done from our home kitchen, and okayed to try by my Dr. Maron.*

We let them freeze in the freezer, popped them out of the mould when hard, and put them in a plastic bag in the fridge until I needed one. This proved to work for pain and not have the "high" effect that I had experienced taking it orally. Eventually, it slowly stopped working because my body adapts to medications and always requires a higher dose (which I was not willing to do).

November came and went and so did my classes. I was making it to classes but I wasn't able to do much else. I was so tired. If I'd have a flare it took me days of extreme fatigue to recover. I usually didn't make it to commuter care groups for games, snacks and fun and I started to feel like a bad wife. I got up in the morning and made it to classes but once that was done I went home to eat and go to sleep. Jason would come in eventually to wake me so I could start on homework and it would be up to him to make supper as I did homework from our bed. (sometimes with my heating pad on high) I felt like a bad wife once again as I wasn't able to do much cleaning, cooking or going out with friends.

Jason worked at his small desk in the living/dining room and came instantly to any text that I sent him saying I needed something. I cried many nights thinking that he deserved better and that I was sorry I was making his life harder, but he was always patient and never saw it that way. People at school told me that our relationship inspired them to see how caring, selfless and servant hearted Jason was to me. And that is pretty much how the rest of the school year went; me doing very little and Jason doing lots.

On April 28, 2018 I walked down another aisle, signifying another accomplishment. I had walked the aisles we (my family) all thought I may never walk because of my health. The aisle at high school graduation, the aisle of my wedding, and this day was the aisle of college grad! I did it with a proud smile on my face as my name was called and I walked on stage to take my three year Bachelor of Arts with a Focus in Counselling diploma.

I walked that stage with my giraffe slippers on my feet as that was how people usually saw me the times I would sit in the student centre for a change of scenery and to see my peers. It was also to show that I didn't lose my spunky personality through the days of pain. With Jason by my side, my friends behind me, and Jesus surrounding me, I graduated!!!!!!

Bonus Material:

SBC Year 3 Courses: Semester 1 - World Religions, Genesis, Counselling: Depression and Anger, Wisdom Literature, and Faith and Science. Semester 2 - Prayer, Urban Missions, Galatians - Philemon, Hebrews, Ethics and Christian Studies Seminar.

Chapter 12: Entering the Real world (Age 21, 2018)

After graduating, Jason and I had two days before we would get possession of the house we had purchased. We packed up our small little apartment on the school campus and moved back to where our families live. We lived in my old basement room for two days, and on May 1, 2018 we got possession of our first house! Both our families helped us unpack and sort things into the different rooms. We couldn't believe how "big" it was compared to our last place. Our house is 1200 square feet compared to our campus apartment of 350 square feet.

After a week of sorting our belongings, Hershey was able to come and live with us. Hershey had missed me a lot when I was in school. We only saw each other some weekends. I became very grateful that he moved in with us, because I had more adeno pain flare ups due to the stress of working on the final papers, doing exams, graduating college, saying bye to all the new friends, moving into my parent's basement for two days and finally moving into our new place. I was so busy and stressed that my flare ups and fatigue didn't allow me to work for the first two months. (Having stress causes endo/ adeno woman to have more flare ups due to tightening muscles.)

Jason, thankfully, found a job right away building wooden crates and he was supportive of me staying home to just rest and heal. During these two months I was however able to join Jason's parents' ministry that translates music, devotionals and stories to Low German and sends it to the struggling places needing God in Central and South America.

To take a load off of my mother-in-law's back I started writing the children's devotionals for her. This helped her not have to think of all the stories herself and would only have to translate them into German (as I don't know German). This was the one way I felt productive, not totally useless, and could help Jason out with the finances. I was able to do this from bed and when I felt up to it on my own time. I had no specific work hours.

Due to not being able to work a full time job, I would go to the clinic and explain my case to a doctor. There was a nurse practitioner working that day who listened to my story. He told me, "You have a good chance of getting disability because you have tried everything including two out of country surgeries, all the most "intense" painkillers and then some."

He filled out the paperwork and sent it away and months later I heard back that I was denied because, "If you can walk, talk, hear, and see, then you are not disabled," (short form of what the denial letter said).

We were able to get to know our neighbours on both sides of our home and learned that we had gone to school with them. Jason knew the ones on the West and I had gone to school with the ones of the East. I began talking to Kris (the East neighbour) about life. In high school we were not close friends but we knew of each other.

She told me about her marriage and it turned out I knew her husband, also from high school. I met her little son and played with him until he drooled on me (I wasn't used to kids). I would spend many days going down to her place to visit. We were both home and not employed. We became close through our visits and she would continue to support me in my journey with my health issues.

In June, I went to visit my Gynaecologist in Winnipeg. My adeno flare ups were coming on more often and were getting more painful so I wanted to see if the doctor had any suggestions for me. He asked questions and typed on his computer. "This definitely sounds like a flare up due to stress. But since you have adenomyosis, the more you have these painful flares the more it is spreading, which means the slimmer your chances are to have children." He explained that the only way to get rid of adenomyosis, is to remove the entire uterus (hysterectomy).

In Canada, the recommendation is that you should be over the age of forty or have had children of your own. Why? The thinking by doctors is that they don't want to deprive women of the chance of having children, even though it should be the woman's choice. This was hard news to hear. He was pretty much saying "have children now or possibly never have them." And never having them meant I may have to suffer many years in pain until around forty and only then would I be able to get a hysterectomy.

I came home and told Jason the news. Many evenings and nights we would cry or just sit and pray asking God what to do. "If we have children now, we won't have a life," Jason said.

"I'm in bed all day with pain and I can't work. I already don't have a life. And this is one step closer to getting the surgery I need for this pain." I said. When we got married, not even a year ago, we talked about wanting to wait about five years to have children. This kind of talk felt like a now or never situation and decisions had to be made.

Finally at the end of that month, (I think June) we agreed that after our one-year anniversary we could start trying. We both sat there not smiling or thrilled about this. I had learned not to get excited about things that may or may not happen in order to save my heart from more heart breaks. We didn't at all feel ready for this, and it felt like the disease was literally pushing us into it.

In July my health improved a little and I got a job. I was already known at the recycling depot so I returned there to see if there were any job openings available. I applied and got a job in Supported Independent Living. The shifts were only 1-5 hours long. I could do this job because there was no heavy lifting, physical activity, and not too many hours to push through.

We celebrated our one-year Anniversary, August 11, 2018. We went to Winnipeg to celebrate. I had planned to do things Jason had never done before. We laughed, and felt worry free as we played indoor glow in the dark mini golf, and got our nails done at an oriental nail place (Jason needs me to note that he did not get polish of any kind). We then concluded our date by watching a movie in the theatre and headed home to relieve my parents from dog sitting!

An anniversary gift I gave to Jason was that I would sit through the Lord of the Rings...all of them! Over the next few days as I watched trying hard not to fall asleep, a quote came up. Many people know this quote but it struck me because of the situation with my health issues over the years.

Sam says to Frodo, "It's like in the great stories, Mr. Frodo. The ones that really mattered. Full of darkness and danger they were. And sometimes you didn't want to know the end. Because how could the end be happy? How could the world go back to the way it was when so much bad had happened? But in the end, it's only a passing thing, this shadow. Even darkness must pass. A new day will come. And when the sun shines it will shine out the clearer. These were the stories that stayed with you. That meant something, even if you were too small to understand why. But I think, Mr. Frodo, I do understand. I know now. Folk in those stories had lots of chances of turning back, only they didn't. They kept going, because they were holding onto something. That there is some good in this world, and it's worth fighting for."

To most this quote may mean nothing, but I've said it to others who have chronic pain, and they agree that it expresses the hard journey but that there's still a reason that they keep pushing forward. This reason is because there is still something worth fighting for in the midst of all the pain and all the darkness.

Our one-year anniversary was complete. August 11 had come and gone. And as planned we began trying to conceive. I kept working at my part time job despite random pain attacks from my adenomyosis.

Chapter 13: Two Lines
(Age 21, September 2018-Now)

After our one year anniversary, I went off birth control. I found it harder to go to work because of this choice. My fatigue and brain fog seemed to be through the roof and my cramping Adeno pain was unrelenting. I guessed it had something to do with being off birth control and I knew that if this was the new me, I would never be able to hold down even my part time job.

Knowing I was denied disability last time; possibly because a nurse practitioner filled out the papers instead of a doctor, I went to the clinic and asked if there was any way I could be on disability of some sort. As I didn't have a family doctor at this time, a receptionist suggested I get an appointment with a doctor who has an interest in chronic pain patients. They suggested I see Dr. Theo.*

I sat down with him and explained my case. I asked him to look at my chart and see if he could write a disability form to be sent in. "This just doesn't seem right," he said. "You are a twenty-one-year-old girl, how can you be asking for disability? Don't you feel horrible that you have to be seeking disability?" I sighed seeing this would be a struggle to have the doctor write this note. "Yes. It feels awful that I'm married and I can't support my family, but I know myself best and I know that I can't work and stay pain free or be "healthy" at the same time. Please just help me."

He was not going to give in that easily and said that part of the issue with people who experience chronic pain is that they let depression or their mindset make their pain worse. He explained how he had created his own Chronic Pain Assessment form, which he liked to use on chronic pain patients, to help see the whole picture from childhood, through to adulthood. He liked to see their past doctor visits, past surgeries, and any medications they've tried and then maybe he would be able to see something that the patient could try.

I forced a smile and said, "Let's get to it."

"Oh no, no, this is going to take four appointments, each an hour long at least." I was not happy. I would have to sit through long appointments once again in my pain and my brain fogged state. As life continued, that is exactly what we did over the next two to three months. I had my first appointment in September and tried my best to go to my appointments open minded to hammer out as many questions and answers as I could, so that this would not have to take so long. We started by looking over my childhood; whether there were traumas, information about my family and extended families health problems etc. I didn't see the point in this, but he thought it very important to have a *full* overview of my entire life.

This was a hard section for me to recall answers about this time; as Lupron had wiped my memory of most everything from those times. So technically, I did finish that section as fast as I wanted! Our appointment ended with one final question. "What are your current dreams and goals for yourself." Oh, if I had a dollar for every time someone asked me that stupid question...I would be rich. It's not that it's a bad question to ask, but when you're asking someone in chronic pain, they don't have dreams because their pain is their only focus. Their only goal/dream is to be pain free.

I looked this doctor straight in the eyes and said, "I had only one dream. And this last February my husband made it come true. I had always wanted to pet a giraffe, a real one. We went to Florida, to Busch Gardens and we were able to pet, and feed a giraffe. If I die tomorrow, my life would be complete by simply finding me the perfect man and being able to pet a giraffe."

He smiled genuinely and typed out my response as I sat there smiling and recalling that wonderful trip. "And your goals in life?"

"I want what any chronic pain person wants. I want to be well. And right now, for my adenomyosis I need a hysterectomy but I am too young. Therefore, my gynaecologist suggested that Jason and I should have a child so that I can have my hysterectomy procedure right after. And that is my current goal." He explained how shocked he was to hear that a twenty-one-year-old had such a big decision on her hands to deal with. He took down his notes and we ended the session.

In the last week of September, my health started to crash. I had severe pain on one side of my abdomen or the other. I assumed these were my ovaries trying to produce my period because I was late. Being late didn't surprise me, nothing about my periods were ever normal and I had just gone off birth control the month before. Two days in a row, at night, I went into the hospital and was given morphine and gravol and sent home to sleep it off. On the second trip I happened to run into a nurse I used to see regularly. I had been away at school so he hadn't seen me in a number of years. "Hey, how have you been doing," he asked me cheerfully. We knew each other by name.

"Well my pain is up and down."

"Shoot, I thought it had gotten better because I haven't seen you for a long time."

"I was just away at college," I replied. "I'm surprised you remember me!" He laughed.

"You were in here every week...I couldn't forget that sad red head who looked to be suffering so much." He tested my temperature and other things in the triage area and we continued talking.

"I'm married now," I informed him. "*Heyyy* congrats!!" He was genuinely happy for me. "Did the doctors ever figure out your problem?"

"Yes," I replied, "at the end of grade 12, I had surgery in Mexico and another one out in California in 2016. I had surgeries for endometriosis. I'm still left with adenomyosis but that will get fixed eventually with a hysterectomy."

I was so thankful to be able to share my story with him and he listened intently, and wanted to learn more. This was what I was wanting for both woman suffering and health care professionals to learn about this disease. It had taken me five years to get diagnosed (which feels like a lifetime) but the average is actually seven years. That is simply *too long*. We had a good chat despite my pain, and he wished me the best as I went to wait in the waiting room.

I was finally called into the treatment room. I explained my situation with adenomyosis and that I just needed morphine and gravol and I could go home, sleep it off and deal with it. The doctor looked over my chart then asked, "Are you possibly pregnant?"

"Probably not." I replied. "OK we'll give you morphine and then get a pregnancy test done just to confirm."

"Sure." I got the pain and nausea medications I needed, and later the nurse sent me home, as I was getting very tired. I just got up on my driveway when my phone rang. The doctor apologized for the nurse who had sent me home so quickly. He told me that he had actually wanted me to do the pregnancy test immediately. I assured him I was probably not pregnant. He said he would still like for me to take an at home pregnancy test to confirm my status, as I had been given extensive pain medication.

I had one pregnancy test at home. At our wedding, Reese had been the MC and he surprised us with a gift basket containing orange items (because I hate orange). There was everything from orange napkins to an orange box of cereal. Even the reusable grocery bag was orange. Reese said "Oops, how did this get in there?" and pulled out a pink pregnancy test. Everyone roared with laughter. It was a great memory and now, I was actually going to use it.

The next day I informed Jason of my hospital trip and that I was fine. He didn't like it when I wouldn't wake him so he could take me but I always felt bad as he slept so peacefully. That was all I told him about the appointment and off to work he went. I took out the test. I felt bad having to waste it. This was going to be pointless. I waited and read the box. Two lines = pregnant. One line means you are not pregnant.

I asked my neighbour Kris if she could look on Facebook because I sent her a picture of the test and didn't know how to read it. When I sent the picture she replied, "THAT'S CLEARLY TWO LINES! CONGRATS YOU'RE PREGNANT!!!!"

No. No. NO. This is not happening. It's wrong. It's from a dollar store. It's wrong. So I jumped in my car and went to the clinic. I waited to see a doctor but everyone in the waiting room was told that the urgent care doctor was called in to the hospital to help assist in an emergency and wouldn't be back till later. I drove to my mom's house and threw my arms around her. I cried and cried. "This isn't happening," I told her. I showed her the test and she was surprised!

"Teya why are you sad, I thought this is what you wanted?" I told her that I didn't think it would happen, let alone happen this fast. Other endo girls wait years to get pregnant, and some never do. My mom and I waited together until we thought the doctor would be back in the walk in clinic. We went to the clinic again. Dr. Adams* was there.

I explained to him the pain I was having on my sides, by my ovaries and also that I had taken an at home test that showed I was pregnant. The doctor sent me to the lab to check if I had a bladder infection. He also seemed to be concerned that I could be having an ectopic pregnancy considering my health issues. The lab technician was a friend of my mom and was always concerned with my health, often asking my mom how I was doing. I asked if I could also have a pregnancy test done too and she said she would sneak it in for me. I stood talking to her about how I came to this point of possibly being pregnant and waited for the results.

The results came back positive for pregnancy and negative for bladder infection. The doctor decided it was important to have this investigated further and sent me to the hospital right away to have an ultrasound. He wanted to determine if my pain was because the baby could be an ectopic pregnancy (stuck in my fallopian tube) or whether this was just part of my chronic pain condition. I was thankful for this quick response and help from this doctor, both for me and my unborn baby.

By this time, Jason was just done work for the day, so I went to pick him up. I explained my eventful morning but neither of us said anything after that. It was surreal to both of us. That evening, October 2, we saw the ultrasound report. It showed that there was something (possibly a fluid pocket) or a baby, and it was positioned in the uterus, not in the tubes. It looked to be 4 weeks and 6 days along. My blood work, also taken at that appointment, was not showing the correct levels for a pregnancy, so I was asked to come back in one week to have all the blood tests redone.

We returned to my parent's house that evening and told them the latest news. When Reese got home, I wanted to have some fun telling him about our news. I looked at him and asked, "So when I walked in, dad said I looked so bloated I looked pregnant. I want your opinion because you're the most honest person I know. Do I look pregnant?" I pulled aside my sweater to reveal my bloated/ slightly pregnant looking stomach.

He looked for a while and thought and then said, "No I don't think so."

Then I said, "You're sure? I want your honest opinion." He gave the same answer. Then I took his pregnancy test out of my back pocket and tossed it on his lap. "Well, I am."

He looked up, "Seriously?"

"Yep and it's the test from the wedding." He was surprised but smiled and congratulated us. Then we phoned Jason's parents and told them the news as well. They were thrilled for us and so excited that what we had been hoping for had happened so quickly!

During this time, I had my second appointment with Dr. Theo* for my Chronic Pain Assessment form. I informed him that I had been getting worse in health as I could no longer take my painkillers now that I was expecting and that I had such bad morning sickness till three in the afternoon. He was happy to hear I was expecting and made a comment close to, "Well girls with endometriosis issues who get pregnant are pain free then so you're well on your way!"

To which I replied, "*Most*! Not all. And I am doing worse than before, I'm not feeling better." This time the questions were mainly around the misdiagnoses, naming all the specialists I had been to, the surgery in Mexico, the surgery in California, and all medications I had tried. Thank goodness I had decided to bring my medical binder with me to this appointment as it had that kind of information and a long list of all prescriptions I had tried and their side effects.

Upon seeing this organized binder, Dr. Theo* said "that is such a smart idea to keep a binder such as this. It's very responsible for such a young person as yourself." I said thanks and that I felt after all the stuff I had been through I really needed to keep track of things properly.\

On October 6th, my parents left for Germany. My dad had back and neck surgery four years earlier and now needed the artificial discs that had been placed in his neck removed. They had gotten infected with bone eating bacteria. They were going to place titanium cages in its place because bacteria doesn't attach to titanium. They would only be back on the 24th. My mom specified I needed to keep her *very* posted on how I was doing while they were gone.

On October 15, I again went into the hospital due to bad cramps. I had an ultra sound and the results came back. I was 5 weeks 6 days along and there was a baby, and it was definitely in the womb. Everything looked normal. Jason and I went home thrilled and I kept my parents posted all along. The nausea was intense, though I didn't throw up.

Another time I went to the ER due to pain and again ran into yet another nurse at the triage. "You look familiar. I remember you," I said to her. "Yes I was just thinking of you the other day and wondering how you were doing." It felt like the nurses cared more about me then the doctors had back then and I let her know the latest finds in my health journey.

It was time once again to go and see Dr. Theo.* This was now my third Chronic Pain Assessment appointment. I told him I had been doing horrible with pain and nausea. He started by saying he had read over all the notes we had taken and realized that I had actually tried every pill and surgery for this condition. "Yes, I know. During our first meeting I said you won't find something new that will help me because I've tried everything. The best thing you can do for me is to help me fight to get disability for this pain."

"You seem hopeless. I think that maybe your depression and mindset is making your pain worse. I think if we work on your depression that will in turn help your pain a bit. You definitely need that hysterectomy but maybe if we work on your mental state you will be able to at least make it to your job and be a functioning member of society. I would also recommend going to counselling." Inwardly, I smiled to myself as yet another "genius" doctor just told me that fixing depression would fix part of my pain.

"Dr. Theo,*" I began, "Last week I told you about my life up to my current state. I explained that I was stubborn enough to push through college because I wanted to be a Counsellor. I have spent the past three years learning about how to have a healthy mindset, and I took counselling from an experienced counsellor as my practicum to complete my three-year Bachelor of Arts. I have depression, but I have a great mindset. I have depression pills that work and I have worked so long to be able to see joy in my pain and to see that this pain has done more good than bad because it has helped me reach other Endo girls who feel hopeless like I did. I don't need counselling! I need to care for my body which right now means getting disability so I don't have to make my pain worse by pushing through work."

There wasn't much left that he could say, so he ignored my statement, and dismissed me with a new appointment date for our final session.

On the night of November 5-6, I had nine hours of severe cramping pain. I could have woken up Jason and asked him to take me to the hospital but I would try sitting up and then just lay back down from being so nauseous and dizzy and confused. I figured I better just wait till morning. By morning, I knew I needed to go to the hospital.

Jason went off to work as I told him he should, and then I phoned my mom. She was working and informed me she could only take me in at lunch time. I said I would wait but the pain in the morning increased, so I called my grandma to take me in. She happily agreed. I dragged myself out of bed, with my empty ice cream pail - just in case chunks flew -, and waited by the door. She drove me to the hospital and I told her I would just wait and she could go home.

After waiting 2 ½ hours, rocking back and forth on the chair from pain and nausea, and a room full of people watching me crying and shaking, my name was called. I went in and lay on the bed curled up in a ball with my pail beside me. The doctor walked in, and below is what happened:

Dr: "So this is very important. What was the date of your last period?"

Me: "It's never been regular so I'm not sure. It was either the end of August or the first week of September. Around there."

Dr: "So you have no way of checking when it was? When was your last ultrasound?"

Me: "Well yes it's on my calendar at home. I brought my calendar in a few weeks ago and told them the date my last period was and asked them to put it in my chart because I won't remember. So it should be in my chart. And my last ultrasound was on the 15th. I have the report here." I started to get it out of my purse but was interrupted -

Dr: "You seriously don't know?" She then got up and stormed out of the room.

I began to worry about whether I had done something very wrong and if she would come back so I pulled up a blank calendar on my phone and thought through my brain fog. I had been waiting for my period at the end of

September but it was late and I started having pain so I had gone into the ER at the end of September and beginning of October to receive morphine until I got my period to help with the pain (which I thought was my uterus trying to have a period). Therefore, my last period had been a month before that, and it was the last week of August. The Dr. came in with a sticky note and read it off to me saying:

Dr: "OK your last ultrasound was October 15. It said you were 5 weeks 6 days. So you will have your baby June 11. So I calculated it for you and your last period was September 5. Now take a picture of this and keep it with you because this is important stuff to know."

Me: "While you were gone I remembered when my last period was. It was August 22-26. And I have a copy of the ultrasound here."

Dr: "I just told you I looked at it. I don't need to see it again. And your date is wrong because I wrote it down for you. September 5. Now tell me what you have been given for nausea."

Me: "I was given Diclectin for nausea. But I can't use it daily due to my past history, which you probably saw in my folder. When I take medications straight for days, then my body just slowly gets immune to it, till I need a higher dose. So I don't take Diclectin every day, I take it on the days I know I need to make it to work. On the other days when I don't work, I don't take it and I stay in bed or at home and deal with it."

Dr: "OK, so you have a good nausea medication; therefore, if your body rejects it then that's that. Now what did you think I would do for you when you came in here?"

Me: "I hardly slept last night. And I think one reason is because of the pain that I have from my adenomyosis."

Dr: "No you mean endometriosis."

Me: "No, again it's in my chart. I got my endometriosis removed and now I only have adenomyosis and that is what I get my pain from."

Dr: "Oh OK." She looked guilty that she clearly didn't look at my chart. "What were you using for pain before you were pregnant?"

Me: "I was using Oxycotin before I knew I was pregnant. But when I came into the ER in October, the doctor said it was safe to use morphine in the first few months. I can only have Tylenol for other aches and pains, but there's no way that's working because I was on serious pain meds before."

Dr: "No ER doctor would ever tell you it was OK to take morphine! I don't know why you came in today to waste your time and mine because you know all you can have is Tylenol, and other than that you just need to suck it up."

Me: "Are you serious? So you're not going to help me?"

Dr: "No there's nothing I can do for you."

Me: "Can I at least have fluids to help with the cramps and possibly the nausea? Part of the problem is I'm so nauseous I don't eat or drink as much."

Dr: "When you drink water do you throw it up on the spot?"

Me: "No."

Dr: "Then you're not dehydrated so I'm not wasting the fluids on you. Just drink more!"

Me: "You're not going to help me in any way? What am I supposed to do?"

Dr: "I don't know. You just need to suck it up. It was your choice to get pregnant. Now all you can use is Tylenol and if you want to go home and take your Oxycotin it's your choice if you want to kill your baby or not."

Me: "So you are going to discharge me and then my work will say I was fine and I should keep working but I can't because of pain and nausea. How am I supposed to support my family if everyone thinks I'm fine? I can't work, I quit my job a week ago (but said I would stay on till they found my replacement)."

Dr: "That's not my problem. Your family doctor can deal with you." She looked at the chart and took the phone beside her and began calling the clinic.

Me while she was waiting on the phone: "If you won't help me at the hospital what is my family doctor supposed to do to help me?" I was ignored.

Dr: "Yes hi this is Dr. Sammy* from the hospital. I have one of Dr. Matthew's* patients here and she needs an appointment with him tomorrow. What is a time that is open? OK 2:30, thank you. Bye."

Dr: "OK so you can go and tell all this to your family doctor tomorrow at 2:30. Now there are sick people who need this room so you need to leave."

Me: "Are you seriously kicking an eight week pregnant lady out of the ER without helping me?"

She looked at me and said, "Everyone has pain, you just need to suck it up." And walked from the room. {The End}

I did actually write a formal complaint regarding my treatment by her and received a call from the hospital stating that they had talked to the doctor who apologized and admitted she had been in a bad mood. (I would later ask

Dr. Danielson* who would confirm that it was safe to use morphine while pregnant only in the first two trimesters).

During the time waiting for my dad to pick me up from this awful hospital experience, I sat in a big open space by myself. I sat down crying, shaking, holding my pail and feeling absolutely broken. The doctors had not helped me in the past but now I felt they were having a part in killing my baby. If I could not get my pain/Adeno attack managed, it would turn into contractions and I would lose my baby. I was terrified. I let all my emotions flow through tears but tried to stop when an older lady sat down in the waiting room across from me. She saw me crying and our eyes met, "Sorry" I replied to start the conversation.

"No, no...It's OK. Are you alright?" And that was all she had to say to start the epic waterworks again, the ones I couldn't stop no matter how hard I tried. She was concerned and came to sit beside me.

"I was diagnosed a while back with two chronic pain conditions one of them is endometriosis. My husband and I found out I am pregnant now," I smiled at that thought, "which we thought would never happen. But I was told not to let my pain attacks get too bad or I could lose my baby. I came to the ER needing help to stop this long pain attack that has me so nauseous." I showed her my empty pail. "The doctor told me to just suck it up and that it was my choice to get pregnant. She told me that I could go home and take Tylenol as that's all that pregnant woman can have, or I can take my prescription pain-killers and kill my baby, but it's my choice." I couldn't talk anymore. I was so overwhelmed by just that thought of what had just happened to me.

"I'm so sorry," is all she could say; she was stunned. But that's all I wanted to hear. I didn't want someone to use those cheesy lines on me again like, "don't worry you're young you'll get better," or "oh I'll pray for you."

"You know I'm writing a book I am going to get published about my chronic pain journey with this condition. I guess this incident here is just another piece to add to the story. Thank you for being caring. It helps after an incident like this." I wiped some of my tears as she rubbed my back.

"I will be looking for your book. I can tell you have an interesting story to tell!" she was kind and gentle. Then I saw out the window my dad's truck pull up. I thanked her for caring and pointed out my ride home. While I was on the way home, I texted my concerned mother. She was asking what I had been given and if it was working yet.

As it turned out, when I texted my mom, crying about the incident, she happened to be at the clinic with our family doctor, Dr. Matthews*and upon learning of my treatment by Dr. Sammy*, he said he would make room for me at the end of the day. I went in to see him and he gave me such hope. He said he heard how I had been treated at the hospital and was so sorry. He said that there was a number of nausea medications for pregnancy and I could be on four different ones at once if my nausea was that bad!

First is Diclectin, which I was already on. The next would be Ondansetron, which he then prescribed for me. This is used for treating cancer patients who are very nauseous from radiation and chemotherapy but it worked wonders for me. The next one available would be Maxeran and lastly was Gravol. I only needed the first two and then I was able to deal with my nausea (rarely resorting to taking Gravol as well). He also told me to alternate taking one for three days then the other the next three days so my body wouldn't become immune to it. This would be proven to work. I was so thankful for my kind doctor who took the time out of his already busy day to help this first time, pregnant girl. I really needed kindness and hope that day and he was kind enough to give it.

That same month, my mom took me to my gynaecologist in Winnipeg (Dr. Danielson*). I could have taken myself, but we enjoy making it a girl's trip and she enjoys driving and supporting me at my appointments. This one was exciting to walk into. To be able to tell the doctor that Jason and I were pregnant and to see an ultrasound picture again with something that looked less circular and more baby-like on the screen was encouraging.

I told him a shortened version of the latest ER trip with Dr. Sammy* and he was not impressed. He said "if you have pain, it is OK to take morphine in the first two trimesters but not recommended after that." He recommended I should not have gone off my Zoloft (depression meds) because it seemed I needed them (and he was right). I had gone off of them once I found out I was pregnant as I didn't know if it was safe for the baby. Jason had noticed lately, that I was not myself. Nothing ever excited me and I didn't feel "love" towards Jason or Hershey and had no motivation to get out of bed.

The doctor explained that Zoloft was a safe medication during pregnancy and I was thrilled to go back on it. He also sent a referral back to a doctor in my hometown that he trusted to become my "baby-doctor" and take on my case. In the referral letter, he stated that she was to write a letter to the hospital stating it was OK for me to be given morphine once in a while for pain from my Adeno, but only in the first two trimesters. I was thrilled that he was always so caring and I even told him I was in the process of writing this book; which he encouraged me to continue to finish and to publish as a way to help raise awareness. I went home feeling inspired.

During November, I had my last appointment, with Dr. Theo* to complete the Chronic Pain Assessment form. He said he had once again gone over all our previous notes and was excited to see the assessment coming together. I sat patiently, waiting for this session to be done, so I could walk out with my doctor's letter and assessment, send it away and file for disability. At one point during this question answer session he stated, "I just don't feel good about writing a disability letter for someone who's twenty-one. What would you rather have me do?"

I was now frustrated that after months of working on this assessment it was sounding like he wouldn't fill out the forms. "Then you can send me to a different doctor who will help me." I said.

"You've been to many doctors and they are all just as good as me. That is pointless."

I sucked in a deep breath and let it out slowly. "OK. Hold on. That is the dumbest thing I have ever heard," I said in a totally calm voice. "I took Counselling and if I had a client phone me to do marriage counselling for them and I specialized in addictions counselling, I am not going to waste my time, their time, and their money trying to help them in a field I didn't specifically study in. I am going to refer them to a different counsellor who studied marriage counselling so they can get the help they need. You did not study chronic pain and get a degree for it, thus you can still send or refer me to a different doctor who will help me fight for disability."

He too remained calm. "We are done here. I will fill out this disability form and attach our Assessment notes and then there's nothing more I can do to help you."

"Thank you," I replied kindly. I watched him print and sign the government papers and I walked out to a different reception desk to have them mailed away.

Upon coming up to this desk I noticed it was the receptionist who had snarled at me the last time I came to her desk. I felt like she didn't like me very much. "This doctor wants me to give these papers to you to be sent away to the address at the top." She took the papers and noticed it was a form applying for disability and looked up.

"I don't think this is going to work just because you're applying for it again and with a different doctor, this doesn't mean you will receive it." With that she prepped it and put it in her out box. I once again had lots of pain and nausea, and was finding it more and more difficult to work but kept pushing myself to try as they refused my disability request because, "If you can walk fine, talk fine, see fine, and hear fine then you are well enough to work."

On November 27th Jason came along with me to our three months pregnancy appointment. It was just a basic appointment. Once we arrived back home, we talked about our fears and worries. "We got pregnant so fast...I thought it would take many months or even years before it would happen if it even happened at all! Are we ready for this?" I expressed that I was worried I would lose the baby. I didn't want to get my hopes up like I had in the past when I thought new medications or surgery would heal me. This would be even more devastating. We prayed together a lot and talked about the future.

"We wanted to travel before we had children. But I guess we will do that during or after." Jason said.

"Or we just ditch them at the grandparents and off we go!" I said enthusiastically, trying to lighten the mood.

Jason frowned, "We barely leave the driveway and you miss Hershey already...you wouldn't be able to do that." We then made a post about our news and our Facebook world was thrilled for us as many of them had kept up with my health battles for years. We felt prayers coming our way and some people even helped us out by bringing us meals and offering us help in different ways. We felt loved and supported and knew we would be OK, no matter what happened.

The time continued to go by. My first three months of nausea was starting to subside, but new problems arose. I had never weighed over 115 pounds but now I was gaining weight and experiencing lower back problems. I was out of breath quickly when walking stairs as the baby was stealing all my nutrients and it was hard for my body with this extra weight. I felt weak and exhausted all day, and had requested to quit my job but forced myself to work as my replacement was not found. When my replacement would be found, I requested to remain as a casual staff doing shifts as I could.

The first time Jason saw our baby was January 31, 2019. We had an ultrasound and together we held hands and watched the little baby moving around. "It's kicking now, do you feel it?" The ultrasound tech asked. "No...I don't. Should I be able to?" "Usually woman can feel it by twenty weeks." I was twenty-one weeks. This led to some worries. Would I ever be able to feel it? Was my uterus so used to intense pain that I wouldn't be able to feel the soft kicks? Was I normal? (I would later talk to my OBGYN (baby doctor) Dr. Lauren* about these concerns). We took the two ultrasound pictures home and showed our families. We watched their excited faces shine and pointed out features of our baby!

The first time I finally felt something inside me move, was February 10th (the start of twenty-three weeks). This was thrilling for me, and my heart jumped for joy. Tears rolled down my face and I hugged my stomach! I had one hospital trip this month due to experiencing lower back pain and cramps at the same time but the morphine helped. I had always been so skinny, that even though I only gained fifteen pounds (only in my stomach), I was feeling straining in my back, ribs, and ankles. I was on my depression meds and they were working great for me; however, with all the new experiences, life was still a daily battle.

The questions swirled in my head. How can I ever be a good mother if I can't even take care of myself? What if I have too much pain after its born and I can't go to the baby when it's crying? What if I am always too exhausted from my surgeries, pain and chronic fatigue that I can't keep up with my own child's energy? Will Jason be the fun parent and I will be the lame one, always heading off to take naps and not doing all the high energy activities outside with them? All these thoughts piled on top of each other and I shared all of this with Jason and he comforted me.

In February, my replacement was found and I became casual staff. My goal was to get the required 600 hours in order to receive maternity leave benefits from the government. With some research we found that it is often very hard for endo girls to get government funded maternity leave as they can't work enough hours due to pain combined with pregnancy. I, however, wanted to try in order to help my husband out as much as I could with the bills. Being casual staff gave me the ability to still pick up a shift here and there. I started having a lot of pain on the outside of my body instead of the inside.

In April, Dr. Lauren* sent me to prenatal massage, where it was discovered that my pelvic bones were pulling apart already. This restricted me from doing many "normal" things. The back pain and pelvic bones pain were intense and increasing. I experienced many sleepless nights due to an active baby (which is positive but hard on the mommy), but because of scar tissue from previous surgeries, doing simple tasks would often cause a lightning bolt of shooting pain in my abdomen as scar tissue was ripping. This pain only lasted a few seconds but it was a very sharp pain which made simple tasks very difficult or even not possible.

I brought up the idea, with Dr. Lauren*, of being induced early due to the pain I was experiencing with my pregnancy. She encouraged me to hold on till thirty-eight weeks if possible, because the baby's lungs needed that time to develop and she didn't like inducing women, she wanted as natural a birth as possible. Hershey continued to give me comfort, and my mom came down to help me out around my house.

By the end of April I weighed 140 pounds and had worked my 600 hours by picking up numerous casual shifts and achieved my personal goal. Jason and my family were so proud of me. Jason continued to work, and I was still picking up some casual shifts, and together we got more and more excited for the arrival of our "mini me!"

During this time Jason and I began our prenatal classes which were evening classes, once a week, at the hospital. The information was incredibly useful and helped us as a couple feel more confident in this new journey we would be travelling together. But this experience was totally opposite of what I was used too. The teacher mentioned things like, "During your birth, it's all about you. If you feel uncomfortable with a certain nurse or doctor you only have to mention this and you will be given a different one. We want you to be comfortable! It's all about you."

Jason noticed me scoff and I rolled my eyes at him. Really? I have the ability to be 'in charge' of everything just because I'm pregnant and in labour? I so badly wanted to stand up and tell the story of my treatment with Dr. Sammy* at the hospital when I was eight weeks along. By the end of the first few classes,

I was curious how much of the information we were learning would be different for me because of my health complications. At the end of one of the sessions, I privately asked the teacher, "Do you know how much different this information would be for someone going into labour with endometriosis and adenomyosis?"

Her face saddened slightly but there was recognition about the disease. "Well the women with these diseases that I have accompanied during labour say that the disease is more painful than the labour. That's the easy part. But because of adenomyosis, the after birth is the worst. Due to not having a period for nine months there is six weeks of bleeding and the hormones start up again. There will be after pains as the uterus contracts which can be a painful process for most, but might be even more painful for you with the disease inside that muscle. This will most likely be the hardest part for you." I felt so relieved that she was educated on my conditions and was able to give me the information I needed. It really was starting to feel like it might actually be about me and the baby as long as I was in the maternity ward.

Seeing as we were starting a family we decided to apply for a different life insurance policy. It was a lengthy process answering many questions. Jason answered his in only 15 minutes, then the phone was passed to me and I answered them honestly, the process taking me close to 40 minutes. Jason received a letter in the mail that he was accepted for life insurance and a month later I still haven't received mine. Of course, when I got it, I had been denied due to my medical history section.

This was disappointing. Once again I feel there is not enough awareness about this disease. Only on very rare occasions does a woman die from endometriosis, it's chronic pain you live with. The government said I did not have a disability but yet the life insurance says I do have a disability and so they won't cover me. This makes it so hard for Endo girls to live a normal life and that's all we want! It's frustrating and it would be nice if everyone would be on the same page!

May 14th was another routine check up with Dr. Lauren* my OBGYN. She entered the room and asked, "Congrats on being at thirty-six weeks now! How has your back and pelvic pain been since the last time I saw you?"

Right then and there, I broke down crying. "I can't do this. I hurt so bad and my pelvic bones are hurting more and more every day. My prenatal therapist said the muscles or tissues around them are all swollen as well. I can't sleep well, I can hardly sit sometimes, and going to the bathroom is becoming more painful." I was used to just pushing through and trying to look strong for Jason and my family, but I just couldn't do it anymore.

She sat quietly and looked sad and about to cry for me. "I know this is hard and you have done so much better than I thought you would do being pregnant with chronic pain conditions. We want mom and baby to be safe and healthy and that may mean inducing you at thirty-eight weeks."

My heart fluttered in hope and worry. Dr. Lauren* explained how the process would go and the date was set for May 29. Through my flowing tears, my concerns started to arise, "I feel so selfish. I want my baby to have the best chance at life, and have the strongest lungs which means waiting to give birth as close to forty weeks. Is it selfish of me to be induced? Will you make sure my baby is OK?"

She smiled kindly and replied, "I will do all I can to make sure everything goes well. I think your baby will be ready for the world at thirty-eight weeks because of how active your baby is. It seems it has good movement, and probably has strong lungs."

In week thirty-seven of my pregnancy I went for my last prenatal massage appointment. "Have you had any other pain?" she asked before starting.

"No. Just the pain in my pelvic bones has gotten worse."

"Mind if I feel and see what's going on?"

"Go for it."

Through the sheet that covered me and showed my massive tummy she felt around for the pelvic bones. "Oh my goodness. You are so swollen and inflamed that I can't even find your pelvic bones…" This was not surprising to me as I had been having more pain by doing things like turning over in bed, lifting my legs to get tights/pants on or squatting and standing back up. "I guess it's good you are being induced soon!" she said. I smiled and enjoyed the stomach and back massage, and she worked on the pressure points in the feet to help bring on labour.

Week thirty-eight (two days before I was going to be induced) didn't start like the others usually did. I woke up at 7am from Jason's work alarm. Right away I noticed I was nauseous and felt like I had slight period cramps, but thought nothing of it and went down to have breakfast with Jason. I did my normal daily things like errands and then had lunch. Upon going to the bathroom I noted blood in my underwear. I called the hospital to ask if I needed to come in and be checked out. They said if it wasn't much then I was fine but if it continued I should come in and get checked out. While on the phone it continued to increase and I let her know I would be coming in.

At 1:30pm I went to the hospital just to make sure everything was alright. I was instantly hooked up to a stress test machine and told that the baby was fine and not stressed. 2:00pm is when the burning "down below" started and bleeding slowly continued. The nurse decided to check if my cervix was getting softer (sign of early labour). Fingers again went where the sun doesn't shine and the "period cramps" slowly got worse. "Wow, you're 3-4cm dilated!" she said. "You've been having contractions probably since 7am when you woke up."

"*What*?" I asked! The nurse told me that Dr. Lauren* was working now and she would come over to check on me. Dr. Lauren* confirmed I had started early labour and could go home to be more comfortable through the contractions. I texted my mom to come to the hospital as it wasn't urgent enough for Jason to come from work and it would be many hours before actual labour would start. That was my thinking according to prenatal classes which said a first time mom usually labours for twenty-four hours before giving birth.

My mom came and stayed till their testing was done and then she drove me to my house and stayed with me as what felt like bad period cramps slowly got worse. I bathed in hot water to help the cramps and my mom afterwards rubbed my back to try to help. By 4:30 I was having really bad pain, pain that was adenomyosis pain at its worst! Jason arrived shortly after 4:30 and my mom left leaving us to labour on our own. Jason quickly showered and packed the last few of the things we needed and we arrived at the hospital at 5:20pm. At 5:41pm a nurse checked to see if I had dilated any further. "Oh my goodness. I think you're 9cm!" she said.

"No that can't be right." I said surprised and looked at Jason's surprised expression too.

"Oh man, you're almost ready," Jason said.

"We will call Dr. Lauren* back and she will deliver your baby!"

Apparently on receiving the phone call Dr. Lauren* asked two more times "Are you sure she's that far dilated? That was just too fast!" Thankfully she didn't live far and arrived quickly. At 5:45 I requested something for the pain. I tried Nitrous Oxide (Wacky Gas) but it helped nothing for pain and only made my mind not feel quite right. I was determined to try to have no pain meds as your baby is said to be more awake when born and the mom feels more like herself after the birth. My determination slowly started to fade as the pain got worse.

"OK I'll take the next "healthiest" option. Please hurry," I requested. Jason rubbed my tightened hand and stroked my hair encouraging me that it was almost done. At 6:12pm they had just gotten the IV in my hand to start Fentanyl for my pain. Just as they were getting ready to insert the pain medication I announced loudly, "I need to push! Quickly give me the pain stuff!"

"No no, we can't now you're in labour!" the nurse said. Four nurses gathered around Dr. Lauren* and encouraged me to push and breath. At 6:31pm our baby was born. Jason and I looked into each other's eyes with tears on our faces as we saw a baby being held up for us to see. That was ours!

"It's a girl!" Dr. Lauren* said. At that point all the worries I had about having a girl who may get endo faded. I was just so thankful we had a safe delivery and that it was *done*! At two weeks early on May 27th, almost 20 inches long, and weighing 6 pounds 9 ounces we felt overjoyed to name her Soren Fiella Friesen!

The next three days I was kept in the hospital. Soren was doing great, but I was not. Because of my adenomyosis (so we thought) I continued to bleed and pass orange sized blood clots. I got weaker, paler, fainter and dizzier. The day after Soren's birth (May 28th), my hemoglobin levels were checked early in the morning as too much blood was being lost. It came back at sixty-seven and should be around 120. They checked these levels again in the late evening the same day and it came back at sixty-six.

Soren was great, very quiet and slept pretty much the entire first twenty-four hours of her life, thus giving me time to try to recover. Because of her tiredness from the delivery and her constant sleeping she dropped to 5 pounds 9 ounces, but the doctors weren't worried yet. Thankfully, she also blessed me with catching onto breastfeeding quickly.

May 29th Soren's weight was checked again and had bounced back up to 6 pounds 2 ounces (the nurses commented on how they have never seen a weight jump like that before from breastfeeding and were very pleased). Dr.

Lauren* was really monitoring my case and suggested an iron infusion to try to help boost my energy levels. For an hour I lay in bed watching the IV line drip the iron that I hoped would help raise my energy level. A little while later I was given a blood transfusion which was a two hour process.

The whole time I prayed and thanked God that my baby was at least safe and healthy and thankful it was me going through this and not her. The nurses were *incredible* (compared to my experiences in the ER). The prenatal class teacher had it right. It really is all about you, serving you, and what you need. Finally, late that evening I had enough energy to go to whimpering Soren myself instead of having to push my call button and have the nurse care for her. I got up not feeling too shaky and walked over to the transparent container that she lay in. Her blue eyes shining up at me. I shed some tears of happiness and joy as I changed my first diaper.

May 30th my blood levels were checked again and came back at seventy-one. That was better and satisfied Dr. Lauren* that I was on my way up. Soren was weighed and was now 6 pounds 3 ounces showing she was gaining weight not losing weight! Finally, just before supper we were discharged. Jason strapped our little bundle of joy in the car seat and with smiles on our faces we headed home to show Soren her new house.

Over the next few weeks my blood levels continued to slowly rise. I did have to take it easy as certain tasks still made me weak or shaky. Soren never really cries (so far) so I have had to set alarms every three hours to get up at night to feed her. She has truly been an angel given to us from God. I have already spent countless hours praying for Soren that God's will would be done in her life. If it is His will that she too have the disease and trials that come with endo, I pray that she would have the bravery and courage to never give up.

I pray for us as parents, if she does get endo that we would be the cheerleaders she needs to encourage her to keep pushing even in times when giving up would be so much easier. I also pray to God that if it's His will that he bless her with good health that He grant her empathy to feel others struggles and pain (something I didn't have before my Endo journey). Day by day, Jason and I pour more love out to Soren and continue to believe there is hope of me being pain free in the future...

***This journey is still ongoing and will probably continue for the rest of my life. I invite anyone who wants to continue with my journey to follow along on my blog. The link is <u>teyaweb.wordpress.com</u> or, if the link has somehow changed overtime, you can also find my blog by searching in Google, "Teya Derksen Battling Chronic Pain," (the blog is under my maiden name). On the blog there is a Contact Me page where I will respond to any emails in a timely fashion! If my journey sounds like that of someone you know, please pass on my information or this book so they can find hope and possibly receive the treatment I did to be endo pain free!

Chapter 14: Completing the Puzzle and Seeing the Whole Picture (Written by my family)

Evelyn Derksen: Teya's Mom

Thank You -

To Jesus Christ: for bringing us through one of the toughest times of our lives.

To doctors: who ordered tests and believed in my girl's pain. You will never know how much I appreciate your help and concern.

To Friends: for your support both through prayers, kind words and finances which have been a great help. Many days when we felt we were at the bottom of the valley, your kind words or messages were just what we needed to help us climb out of the valley and continue our climb up the mountain.

My Goal   for writing this chapter, and also for helping Teya write this book, is to raise awareness about how difficult this disease is; but not to belittle anyone. My aim is to inspire professionals in seeking out the latest facts about this disease and in turn to be able to help diagnose Endo patients more quickly. Also, for professionals to recognize when an Endo specialist is required in the care of an Endo patient.

My Prayer - is for quicker diagnoses and for Endo and Adeno to be recognized as a disability by our government. For our government: to also seek out more Endo specialists for Manitoba or at least in Canada, so that girls/women can get the help they so desperately need.

Teya was born a spunky redhead, with so much life and energy. She always kept us hopping. She had a great sense of humour, loved to help us with chores and loved to have sleepovers with her brother. They really loved each other and still do. Little did we know back then, that this carefree loving spirit would leave us in only a few short years and be replaced by a child crying night after night, day after day, and asking God if she could die.

Some of you may wonder - what is it like to have a daughter who is going through endometriosis? How did you handle this? Where did you go for help? Did you always believe she had a disease/pain? I would like to write to a variety of people, and hopefully in the process answer some of these questions.

To Health Care Professionals:

If you are in the healthcare field; such as a doctor, nurse or even a receptionist at a clinic, I have one piece of advice for you. Please treat every person with respect - whether you believe them or not. Try to help patients by listening, and I mean *really listening*. Women feel so hopeless and worthless when they are told, "no you don't have this pain you are describing, it's all in your head." This is what so many women hear time and time again and this has led to depression, and many suicides in young woman. I do not say this to make anyone in our past feel bad. We want to thank every health care professional for any tests ordered, any love shown and for the times they gave us hope.

There's one story I remember about someone feeling no hope. I recall being on an Endo site and seeing this young woman (twenty-years-old) talking about her pain and trying to find someone to believe her and her condition. I'll call her Lynn.* I felt so sad for her that I started to write her and talk about what had all helped Teya. I told her about medications Teya had tried, and what had helped to relieve a little of her pain, and what had not. I told her about certain doctors that had been understanding but since I didn't know any of the doctors in B.C, I couldn't recommend any of them to her. I encouraged her not to give up, but to keep searching.

I told her about Teya's operation in Mexico and then California and how getting Endo excised was the best thing we could have done for Teya. She asked if she could call me. She called me from B.C and as we talked, my heart was breaking for this young girl in search of HOPE. She needed someone to believe her and needed a way to get to a doctor who would believe her, and that could help her. I felt extremely close to her as I thought of my daughter and all that she had been through. For many days I prayed for her and asked Jesus to make a way for her to get the healing she needed. One day I opened up my iPad, and there on the same Endo site I saw.… "Rest in Peace Lynn.*" My heart dropped! Could this be the same girl I had communicated with? If so, what happened?

I messaged around trying to find out if this was the girl from B.C. I found someone who knew the girl and the situation and she told me that Lynn* had in fact taken her life. I believe the lack of hope was too much to bear. She needed support around her and she just wasn't able to handle this any longer. PLEASE GIVE HOPE. These are not just girls looking for attention. These are real human beings suffering with a disease that is rated as one out of the ten most painful diseases out there. They don't look sick on the outside so it is hard to believe them, but if they are missing life events day after day, you know they are not faking it. It's real!

How can a doctor give hope? Listen, tell them you believe them, and if you can't say that, then tell them you would like to confer with a colleague, or ask a colleague to come into the room in hopes that they understand what this pain is all about. Tell them you will research what this type of pain could be coming from. This leaves the patient feeling *hopeful* and not *hopeless*. There is a huge difference in these two feelings for a patient with this condition. It literally could mean life or death!

We are very understanding as your patient when you say, "I really don't know." How could you know everything, you are only human yourself. We understand that with so many diseases out there, the amount of time spent learning about each disease is minimal. However, don't leave it there. Reassure them you will continue to research the problem and strive to make this the best outcome you can for this patient. It is amazing when you start to research the kind of information you will find. You will hear about the latest medica tions and techniques.

Don't just rely on your medical school training, after all, things are evolving and with the research that many endometriosis specialists are doing, they are discovering new facts about this disease daily. They are also finding that a lot of things taught in the textbooks are very inaccurate. One example is the recommendation to have a baby and then you will be Endo free.

I say this to all healthcare professionals with the utmost respect. Your job is not easy, and I know that. I just want all these Endo girls and woman to be understood, so treatment can begin a lot sooner than the average of 7-10 years.

Parents:

You know your children best. If you see that day after day your child complains of pain, don't give up on getting the best help you can for your child. Listen to your child. Support your child by making them as comfortable as possible. Set up doctor appointments and make sure you are there to help them make decisions. Let them know you are in this together and you'll never leave them alone with this condition, as long as you live. Even if your daughter is an adult, this support is a *must*.

My daughter was always sad when another birthday approached and I finally figured out why. She was so scared that when she became an adult she would be expected to make all these hard decisions on her own. She didn't feel sure she could succeed at life. On her eighteenth birthday she broke down crying, saying she couldn't live life like this on her own. I realized then how much support she needed and I let her know we were in this together till the end.

When a girl is in this much pain, her mind will not always function as it should, due to intense brain fog. Answering simple questions like: "have you tried this type of birth control before? Did it help with your pain?" will be super tough for them to recall. I kept a pain journal for a while which really helped me answer a lot of questions about medications, pain levels and whether we wanted to try this route again.

When Teya got married, I had compiled a binder of all Teya's test result papers, a list of medications she had been on, what had worked for her and what didn't, side effects and doctor appointment notes which I then gave to her husband and herself. This gave them the confidence they needed to continue this journey together. To this day she takes this binder to her appointments and now feels she can tackle her own health with the knowledge that I am still here for her if at any time she needs me.

If you choose to compile a binder (which I highly recommend), get as many test results from your clinic as possible; blood-work, MRI's, Ultrasounds etc. This will help you keep track of dates when tests where run and you are also able to research the findings first hand. This could also be helpful if you do choose to see a doctor that isn't in your area. This gives them a glimpse into what has already been tried and what the outcome has been. This could speed up your treatment, as the doctor doesn't have to wait for these records to be sent to their clinic first. And sometimes, you find things in the results that the doctor has missed.

Be a proactive parent. Don't worry about getting doctors/people who don't understand. You are there to advocate for your child. It is your right and I believe your mission; after all, did God not entrust this precious child to you? When your child becomes an adult living with Endo and if they still want your help, your child should request to have your name put on their chart. This will allow you to sit in on their appointments, access to ask questions about your child's treatment, and you can advocate for them.

We had an incident where I was called an overbearing mom. I was listed on my daughters chart, and yet this was not checked when I wanted information. If this person had just looked at the chart, she would have seen that I was listed as an advocate and wouldn't have needed to call me names. I told her I was listed and suddenly she felt bad. It is your right to request information, if you are listed, so don't let others tell you differently.

There was a time where I really felt I was at my lowest. I felt like I had to keep everything together for my family. My husband supported me as much as he could but I knew that if I were to get help for Teya, I would have to do the research. One day as I was putting away the vacuum cleaner away in the closet and had been thinking about Teya's pain, my husband and his health issues, my mom who had at the time been diagnosed with Alzheimer's and was starting to fade. It felt like my whole world was spinning and I couldn't stop it. I was hanging up the hose and I broke down sobbing, with everything in me. I couldn't look strong for another moment.

I silently shouted at God, asking Him for some kind of relief. Asking Him how I was to carry all of this on my shoulders? I was probably in that closet a good 15 minutes and was so thankful no one came to find me at that time. When I emerged, I had a renewed strength, which could only be from God and I was ready to tackle this crumbing situation once again. I felt I had HOPE again. Somehow, I knew things would be OK.

A few weeks later, I sat in church and was praying as the music was playing. I was praying that somehow God would make it clear to me that things would be OK. Suddenly, I can only describe this as God's voice, I heard the words "Bible School" (this being while Teya was still in high school). Before I could even process what I had just heard a feeling of warmth washed over me and I couldn't help but smile. I knew instantly that I had heard God's voice. That something wonderful would happen in Bible School and that everything would be OK. God had a plan and it was a wonderful one. Teya grew so much as a person there, learned how on her own to deal with her health issues, and met her wonderful and supportive husband who we thank God for every day!

Over the past years I've heard some compliments such as, "You're such a strong person," "Teya was given the right mom," or "Your family is lucky to have you." I've also been told not such helpful things like, "You're an overbearing mother and it's time to let your daughter grow up," or "You need counselling yourself," and so on. I probably do need counselling after those many tough years.

Have I been overbearing with my daughter's health….you bet! I've been forced to be. When others didn't take her pain seriously, I had no choice but to step in. I did what God asked me to do, take care of my family. Why would I leave when I was needed the most? "Do unto others as you would have them do unto you." I am in the process of trying to forgive the negative comments that have been said to me and my daughter. I try to remind myself that people have not walked in our shoes. God forgives and requires me to do the same.

ENDOMETRIOSIS:

I love it when people ask what it feels like to have Endo. I don't have Endo but I love to explain it this way as I think this is the best explanation I have heard.

Imagine having blisters all over your pelvis and on your different organs. They pop, puss and hurt. This sequence leads to the formation of adhesions. These adhesions can string your organs together and pull them out of place, attaching them one to the other. When your menstrual cycle is coming, these blisters fill with blood and pop. Now they are even more painful. Your organs swell and the pulling pain is intense.

One specialist's description to a male was put in this word picture. "Imagine your male anatomy stapled to your leg and then you are told you need to run a mile, and do everyday life. That is the intensity of what kind of pain an Endo woman feels. Now imagine that it doesn't only last for a few minutes, it can last for weeks, and this whole time people are telling you your pain isn't real and you should just push through. Or maybe yoga will help."

ADENOMYOSIS:

Adeno is exactly the same idea; however, these blisters are contained in the muscle that surrounds the inside of the uterus. They fill with blood and sometimes pop, other times they harden. It is a super painful condition only cured with a hysterectomy. People wonder why it is that an Endo specialist is needed to remove this disease and not just a gynaecologist?

Imagine for a minute you are told you have a cancerous tumour. A general surgeon says he will remove it and that you don't need to go to the cancer specialist. You know the general surgeon has done a lot of operations on people with great success; however, he does many different kinds of operations per day and does not specialize in cancer operations. You would wonder would he know exactly what to remove? Would he recognize if he spotted more cancer than just the tumour? Wouldn't you feel better going to a cancer specialist who just removes cancerous tumours day after day? After all, that is his specialty.

Endo specialists, specialize in Endo. They know the best techniques, how to recognize all the forms of this disease, the latest research on the disease and they understand the best way to remove it; in order to not have Endo return. That is why we went to see Endo specialists and we were not just happy to let a gynaecologist do Teya's surgery. We wanted to have the greatest chance that she would remain Endo free her whole life.

When Teya began having her menstrual cycle, she lost a lot of blood. I could physically see that her little body was having a hard time with her periods. Watching the pain she was experiencing was a whole different issue. You see the symptoms of pain; such as holding her stomach in a crunched over position, vomiting as the pain increases, passing out from the pain etc. But the pain, you *can not* see.

In the beginning, I did question whether Teya's pain was really so bad when she first got the pain attacks. Before long, I could see it coming without her telling me. I knew then that this was for real. I started to watch her closely and could soon see that I had it completely backwards. Her pain was worse than she was telling me and she was pretending it was better than it was! Then she'd pass out, or vomit, and I would know it was worse than she let on. People with chronic pain are faking being well, *not* faking being sick. They don't want to be sick. They want a life too.

A question I'm often asked is: 'how did you research this disease?' The first thing I did was to get attached to Endo groups on Facebook. They are closed groups and you have to be accepted. I had to explain that I wanted to be on this group to get help for my daughter. I was able to connect with women all over the world and see that they were all suffering as well. I felt amazed when reading their stories or hearing their questions.

I couldn't stop reading. I was super excited and ran to share what I had found with Teya. She looked at the Endo site as well and very quickly said, "mom, I can't read this." She had tears in her eyes as she saw so many women just like her. Some were talking about the pain, some sharing about their families, husbands/boyfriends or medical professionals not believing them. She just couldn't take seeing all the devastation that goes along with this disease. I stayed on these sites and was determined not to lose hope. These sites, for me, represented *hope* for the first time in a long time. Here, I found understanding woman and even some very influential doctors giving out advice. I was so excited!

I asked questions, collected information, and learned so many new things. One important difference was between excision surgery and ablation. I learned that the gold standard is excision. I learned that not all Excision Surgeons have the same amount of training, skill level and experience. Some are only able to get the superficial disease, while others are able to remove the deep-rooted endometriosis. I learned the questions to ask a surgeon and that it's OK to question them and find the right treatment for my daughter.

I could go on and on but there is not enough room in this book. I went on the Endo group for Canada and learned that we didn't have an Endo specialist in Manitoba. There were only two doctors recommended as top specialists, one in Toronto and one in B.C. Both of these surgeons had wait times of 2 ½ years, just for the initial appointment and another year wait for the actual surgery. This was very disheartening and not acceptable, in my view. I heard women share stories about trying to go to another province to get care with one of these surgeons only to be told that a gynaecologist in their city were just as qualified.

Doctors didn't understand that in most of the cases where Endo is present that an excision specialist is the best chance for the removal of this disease to lessen the chance of it reoccurring. They were losing hope in getting the best treatment, the only treatment that might actually get rid of Endo. That's when I decided it was time to look outside of Canada, no matter the cost.

Endo is one of the diseases that has no cure. You can never be cured of Endo; however, if you have endo excised by a specialist, who is trained in deep-rooted endometriosis, it is possible for it not to return. The doctor that we took Teya to in California had a very high success rate. To date, Teya is Endo free for three years now. She is just left with adenomyosis only curable through a hysterectomy.

Teya has had a very wonderful and understanding gynaecologist in Winnipeg for the last few years now. He has been an incredible encourager to both of us. Teya was referred to him from the paediatric gynaecologist that she had been seeing. Upon seeing him, I asked him how he could help Teya. He looked at all the treatments she had already tried, and explained that he could do surgery for her.

I asked if it was excision or ablation. He explained that he did both. The bigger pieces were excised and the small "grains of sand" is where he would use ablation. I told him that I meant no disrespect; however, that was not the type of surgery I wanted for my daughter. I wanted full excision by an endometriosis specialist. I told him we had been in communication with Dr. California* and that we were really considering going to see him to have him do the surgery.

"Good for you in researching options for your daughter. He is top of his field. If more women took time to figure out what treatments are all available out there, less women would land up getting to stage 4." I was shocked and asked this gynaecologist if he would still be Teya's doctor when we returned and he said, "of course." To this day I have such respect for this doctor. He has never treated us differently for taking Teya out of country for treatment when so many others do treat us differently now. We feel cared for and loved - it's a nice feeling!

Friends:

What can friends do for an Endo girl? DON'T LEAVE. Stick by your friend. You may not always understand how they are feeling, and it can get very frustrating when they cancel plans with you again, but give grace. They have a very painful condition, and they are very discouraged and likely depressed. They are sad that so many people don't believe them and that they just can't be normal. Just think about this, you only see a glimpse of their condition when you are with them, which is probably an hour or two, while they live with it 24/7.

I have made a few really good friends through this disease. A few have the disease themselves and a few are Endo girls moms. I have enjoyed visiting with them, hearing their stories, and we support each other. There is just nothing like a person who truly understands. The caregivers of all the Endo girls/women also need support. We were blessed to have great family support, friends and church support. Many gave us money towards Teya's surgeries. We are very thankful!

This disease changes the whole family. It was hard to go out for a visit as we would often need to cancel and stay home to care for our daughter. I've even noticed that I've personally changed a lot because of this disease, dealing with my husband's pain issues and my mom's Alzheimer's. I really felt that it was just too much to handle at times. I have medication for anxiety now and find myself not to be as trusting as I used to be. I find it harder to be in crowded areas and tend to enjoy being at home by myself now. These are things I am working on daily.

I've looked at the health struggles of my family like a giant puzzle. We try to place each piece, so we can see the finished picture. Sometimes it takes a long time to find a piece and next time, it's placed in seconds but each piece gives us more of a glimpse of the final product. I often wondered why my husband has had to suffer with headaches for more than twenty-years now and back and neck issues to boot. Then along comes Teya, who has so much pain that can't be diagnosed for five-years and could only be diagnosed by going out of country for help.

The two of them have been able to support each other as they both understand severe pain and understand surgeries. In the midst of all of this, my mom, who was always so kind and truly understanding, a true encourager, passes away. She has left a hole in my heart. Teya has learned so much in supporting others with pain through her own situation. She wants to help people by using methods like counselling and support. Not bad for a girl who didn't have compassion for people before her pain started. Teya has talked about sharing at youth groups and giving inspirational talks to women. I think she could help a lot of people. The puzzle pieces are fitting together and I couldn't be happier. I'm really starting to see the picture and it's a beautiful one!

-Evelyn Derksen

If you are in need of support, or have any questions for me, I encourage you to contact me. 1-204-325-9860 or lonievelynderksen@gmail.com.

Loni Derksen - Teya's Dad

As a Father, I always tried to raise our kids to be independent. As they matured, they were given more and more responsibilities. When Teya became sick, this became more difficult. Some days she did great with putting her dishes in the dishwasher, or wiping the table after eating and then other days she was needing her food served to her in bed and we would take care of the dishes. This is a time when I myself was also dealing with chronic pain issues, so my wife did most of the caring for Teya. At this time, I had dealt with headaches 24/7 for many years. I had my first back surgery to fix a herniated disc but ended up removing it completely years before Teya's issues started but was still dealing with pain.

I focused on going to work to keep my mind off of my own pain. If I would have allowed myself to stop or stay home, all I would think about was the pain. I used work as a coping method to keep my mind off of my pain. I worked a full-time job and ran a small family business on the side.

When I would come home from work and would hear that it had been a tough day for her, I would often go into her room and support her by joking around with her and telling her stories of the day. This would help Teya also get her mind off her pain and therefore she seemed to do a little better in the evenings. It would land up becoming almost a family evening activity; sometimes all four of us lying in her bed and joking around. Humour was another way we used to deal with many of life's issues. This time seemed to bring us closer together because we couldn't make plans with others to go out as we had two people dealing with chronic pain in the house.

I tried not to let my own pain stop me from doing daily duties. I would push through my pain to get things done. Sometimes Teya was lying around and would ask me to get her something. At times I would ask her to get it herself saying, "you have two legs you are able to do it yourself," this often made her upset. I was trying to teach her to work through her pain and never give up, and she took this as if I didn't care about her condition. We clashed for a while, as our thinking was so different in how to deal with our pain situations. This left my wife to mediate between us. I've learned that everyone deals with pain differently.

Our laying around and joking evenings also led to more prayer times. We would spend time asking God to help us both get through another day; sometimes even just another hour, asking Him to give us wisdom in how to deal with our own situations, and give grace for others also dealing with health issues.

For many years this was our life. We both had conditions that the doctors here seemed to have no answers for. We were both on many pain-killers and many other types of medications and there seemed to be no fix in sight. At this time, my mother-in-law was also diagnosed with Alzheimer's and my wife was feeling very overwhelmed. She felt that she had another person to care for and to watch fade away. I was tired of seeing doctors and not finding any solutions. My attitude was that I was done fighting for help because it was pointless. I wasn't suicidal but if I had gotten the news that I had only a few weeks to live, I would have been very at peace and even happy with this.

Teya, on the other hand, became suicidal. She begged God often, to let her die. This began to feel like a very hopeless situation for my wife. When my wife heard me say I was done wasting my time seeing doctors, she started researching surgery in Germany. For me this was simply too much money to spend on myself, but one day she said "how much fun will it be for me to have you sitting in a wheelchair in pain, and have money in the bank. I'd sooner be broke and sit on the back deck drinking ice tea with a healthy husband and be able to work to pay it off."

This made me understand that we would not be spending the money only on my health, but her happiness and my families in the long run as well. In January 2015, we flew to Germany and I had two artificial discs put in my lower back and two in my neck as well as a couple of bone spurs removed. This gave me hope to finally have pain relief. Teya then asked my wife if she could also have surgery? She desperately wanted relief from her pain as well. My wife started to research other places that could possibly help Teya.

Shortly after our Germany trip, my wife found a doctor in Mexico who thought he knew what her problem was and could help her. Teya was finally feeling hopeful. We looked into the cost of this surgery and were surprised the whole trip was only $10500.00. Compared to the Germany surgery this sounded very inexpensive and we decided health was more important than money. We flew to Tijuana, Mexico, only a few months after my surgery and met with the doctor.

During the doctors consult, he did an internal ultrasound and we could all see Teya's uterus contracting as if it had a heart beat. When the doctor inquired about this she said it never stopped. This made her pain a lot more real for me. He agreed she had endometriosis and he was willing to do the required surgery. This made me feel hopeful that she could also have less pain.

The surgery was a great success; however, her pain slowly returned around six months later. Teya became upset that her pain had returned and she questioned why I was doing so well and she wasn't. I had to explain to her that I still had my constant headaches and still had to work smart because my body was not back to how God made it. I was not pain free, just so much better than I had been. I also dealt with this pain differently than Teya. I was thankful for the relief I had gotten and how far I had come. Teya wanted to be 100 percent pain free.

A year after her Mexico surgery, my wife found another doctor. This time the doctor was in California. He would be willing to see if he could help her. My wife was on a mission once again to help Teya. I looked into the cost of this surgery and it was $40,000.00. Again, much less than the Germany surgery but I didn't know where we would get another large amount of money. I was feeling a lot of pressure to provide. This is where my faith needed to come in. God had provided for us this far and I needed to have faith he could do it again. People were kind to us and helped us out with prayers and some donations.

Teya had her surgery in California and this time I had a talk with her and told her not to expect to be pain free, but rather to be thankful for any relief that she would receive. The surgery was a success. This was three years ago and she is still endo free to date. The doctor did however discover she had another problem called adenomyosis (endo in the muscle that surrounds the uterus). This can only get better by removing the uterus. Something she wasn't quite ready for at the time as she was only nineteen.

We were also never sure if she would be granted children with this condition. Thankfully she got married to a great guy almost two-years ago and they are expecting their first child. God has granted us some amazing gifts. If you are a parent of an endo daughter try not to focus on the money that is spent on a surgery. For myself, we were offered no other options here in Canada and for Teya we wanted the best surgery option available and not a band aid fix. When a person has hope and feels better they have a much healthier outlook on life. This is something you can't attach a price tag to. The mountains were at times hard to climb and we stumbled along the way but now looking back we see how far we have come. God is good, all the time.

–Loni Derksen

Reese Derksen: Teya's Brother

I don't remember the first time Teya was sick but I do remember comforting her. Sitting at her bedside telling her that everything was going to be alright; not knowing if it actually would be. She was clearly in pain, which made me uncomfortable. Seeing someone you love go through suffering is never a fun ordeal, and I had always had a very big heart for everyone around me.

Teya had always been my big sister and took her role very seriously. No one was allowed to hurt little brother Reese, except for her. When it came to family matters she reflected the cornerstone approach our mother took; caring for another person when they needed help was priority number one. It didn't matter the scale of the injury, sickness or issue, mom was always devoted to our wellbeing. Teya soaked up these traits and found it in herself to assist others who needed help.

Now she was the one lying in bed, needing my help. I knew it was only right to support her, like she had done so many times for me. I sat with her for a long time, making jokes and chatting about nothing important to distract her mind, until her pain had died down to a minimal. Then I checked to make sure she didn't require anything else before I left. Based off the smile I received, I knew she was thankful for the time I had just spent with her. She knew that her little brother would always be there for her.

I don't remember the 100th time Teya was sick but I do remember leaving the house instead of comforting her. She was currently lying in her bed, screaming about how she wanted to die. She asked if I would end her life, because that would also end the suffering she felt every day. Unfortunately, this wasn't the first time she had asked me to kill her.

Every week the pain seemed to be getting continually worse. This downward spiral had stretched so long I was numb to her suffering. Putting on my headphones I could no longer make out the sobbing wails she was emitting, as my mother attempted to console her. Turning up the volume, I made sure I couldn't hear any noise other than my music as I left the house. It didn't take me long to get outside because I always had a backpack prepared, filled with sketching equipment in case Teya's condition started getting worse. The easiest way to deal with my sister's condition was to not think about it, and I had become skilled at that.

Getting on my bike I usually drove to the same spot every time. This was my happy place. Here I was free to sit alone in silence and create a better world than the one I was residing in. Art had always been a passion for me and having total control over a minuscule portion of life was wonderful. A few years before this I never listened to music. Now I used it as an escape. It was a way to transport myself as far away from my family's health problems as possible. I would always ride my bicycle away from home, but it never took me as far away as music did.

I began creating graffiti art when I was thirteen-years-old. The allure of this art with no rules or limitations allowed me to fill my sketchbook extensively, soaking the page in ink that stank of that signature Sharpie smell. I had heard of people using markers and glue to get high, but this never interested me. Music and art were distracting enough to take my mind off whatever was happening at home right now. The amount of time I spent away from the house was usually dependent on when I thought Teya's pain attack would be over. Usually it would start getting late and I would have to begin packing up.

I never told my parents where or when I was going out, but I figured they had more important matters on their plate anyways. Since Teya became sick her condition ensured that my parents gave her the majority of attention between the two of us. I didn't mind this that much though as I preferred to be alone anyways. It gave me time to think about everything that was going on in life.

On a few rare occasions I would sit in my happy place and cry to myself. I made sure to try and cry here because I didn't want to cry at home. Crying was something I thought of as a weakness, and based off the state of our family there was no room for weakness. I saw emotion as a whole in that way.

Emotion was a vulnerability. Most of life at this point felt depressing, so I no longer wanted to feel. The solution I decided upon was to cut out the large amount of sensitivity I had inherited from my mom. This ensured I could never feel miserable again, because I wouldn't let myself feel anything.

I've gone through some of my old baby photos with my mom before, and unknowingly she always makes the same statement; "you used to be so happy." This single innocent sentence always pierces my heart, and deflates it because I know she's right. When Teya was sick I did not know how to handle it. This paired extremely poorly with my excessive independent mindset, so I never asked for help.

On Wednesday nights I would go to Youth and every week they would ask if anyone had prayer requests for struggles happening in our lives. I knew that my sister was sick in bed, unable to attend school due to an unknown sickness she had. I knew that my dad was at work, because that helped him cope with his pain and provide an income for his crumbling family. I knew that my mom was at home researching illnesses for her undiagnosed daughter, and was almost being crushed by the amount of problems she felt the need to fix in her family member's lives. Yet I never brought it up. I would sit quietly every week, bottling up all the emotions in the hell that was life, and quietly pushed them down as if they didn't exist.

This unhealthy way of dealing with pain gave me a dark outlook on life, and I slowly pulled away from friends and family. I never felt like I had the right to speak up though, since I had no chronic health problems myself, and couldn't truly understand what they were going through. My dad has always been very good at ignoring his pain, and this is something we have both probably taken too far. There is a good and bad way of ignoring pain, and I was good at doing things the bad way.

All these thoughts and feelings are things that I have never actually shared, and I'm only acknowledging them now to myself, years after the darkest times have passed. Only now am I seeing the grotesque mindset I had developed, almost mimicking a robot in the way that I solely operated off logic and reason once I decided emotion was a weakness that I could no longer afford.

Before going to bed one day I was mulling over all my medical issues. I had no chronic pain. I was prescribed no medication. I didn't need to go to the doctor. I had no allergies. I had 20/20 vision. I had perfect hearing. All of this was confusing to me, and I began asking God why He cursed the rest of my family with problems but not me? Why was I getting the special treatment?

I decided I would challenge God to see if he was truly fair. That night I prayed to God, asking for Him to give me cancer so I could be sick too. Usually I tried to think with logic and reason, but I had neither of those in mind when I made my request. I just wanted to be able to identify with my family's struggles, and in some capacity receive the same level of love and affection that I watched Teya receive. I could have just asked my parents for more attention but I felt wrong in doing so without a justified reason, and my independent attitude went against this idea. My parents needed to focus on Teya because she was the sick one.

"I was the perfect child." That's what Teya said about me one time when she was having a severe pain attack. Unfortunately most of my battles had been mental ones, so my battles scars were not nearly as evident as hers. In my head I was fighting my own war, but I just smiled and agreed with her that I was lucky to be "the perfect child."

At the start of her sickness Teya would usually have an attack alongside her period. As Teya's peculiar symptoms began to return, and at seemingly random intervals too, my parents realized that this was not an exclusive issue. Something was wrong with their daughter, and it was recurring. Without knowing how big this problem would eventually become, my parents took the first of many steps towards curing their daughter. The only problem was that we had no idea what specifically we were needing to cure. In order to get a proper answer you need to establish what the problem is first. This led to many trips to the emergency clinic, and an abnormal amount of hospital visits. Teya even kept her hospital check-in bracelet on, due the frequency of visits, which allowed her to more efficiently get help. Some staff already knew her by first name.

Time after time Teya would go to the hospital seeking help and answers. Usually she was given pain killers in an attempt to alleviate some of her suffering, but explanations were never available. This vicious cycle would repeat, with medical professionals being baffled as to why this was occurring. Soon some doctors began to question the legitimacy of her claims. I believe a dose of skepticism is healthy, however we were far past that point. The ignorance some doctors directed at Teya began to be revealed, and my mom was viewing it firsthand. Teya often was unable to properly communicate during these intense pain attacks, so my mom became her guardian angel, conversing between both parties.

I usually didn't want to go with them to the hospital, so my mom or dad would take her. Then they would return with Teya in the evening and share if a doctor had made any amount of progress in diagnosing the mysterious condition. It was rarely good news. Slowly some doctors began to brush her off due to the high frequency of her visits. Her case was a mystery and instead of diving deeper into their patient's issues, they opted to see her as a nuisance instead. From their perspective Teya was a waste of time, and these distractions were not welcome. A few seemed to believe that she was worthy of an academy award in acting with the intense pain she was able to incredibly fabricate.

Some days my mother would come home and tell us that the doctor had informed them that Teya was perfectly well, and she should simply stop pretending to be sick. This dismissive remark made me want to smash the doctor's skull in with a hammer until they screamed in agony, just like I had heard my sister scream, and then I wanted to ask them why they were faking their pain. Unfortunately I had a very creative imagination, which would begin silently conjuring up various ways the doctor could experience the same level of pain Teya was feeling. It would not be obvious to other people that I was angry though, because I would get quieter and distance myself from those around me. I was never a physically violent person, but hearing a medical professional talk about my sister in such a condescending manner made me wish I was.

These angry thoughts did not translate to action though. I didn't talk to anyone about them either. Instead every negative comment made by any doctor, only added to my hatred for the group as a whole. I found it ironic that in our society, doctors symbolized health and compassion. It felt like the very same people that were meant to be protecting my sister were also killing her. This left me with a gaping feeling of hopelessness. Until now I had put total blind faith in our healthcare system. Now that the doctors had refused to even try and help diagnose her, where were we supposed to go?

The unregulated world of medicinal miracles was the only area left. Just like we were doing for my dad's medical condition, we began trying anything and everything that was available. From religious healing to unorthodox practices my parents were at a point of desperation that didn't allow them the luxury of passing up a possible solution. One product was clearly a pyramid scheme, but writing it off before testing was not an option. Like all the other products before, it ended up not being effective at anything but taking our money.

Looking back now, I am thankful for the handful of doctors and medical professionals that did actually care for her. Many of them did believe her pain was real, but were unsure of how to diagnose the issue. A few of them continued to try and provide some sort of answer, long after most had already assumed she was a lost cause. I wish I could recognize who all these human beings were, but I tended to avoid the hospitals and waiting rooms so I never met any of them except for one doctor. The only doctor I met was the one that ended up saving my sister. I never got a chance to tell him this so I'll write it here now:

Thank you for saving my sister. Like the other doctors, you were not perfect because you are human. Unlike the other doctors, that did not give you a reason to abandon my family when we were at the point of breaking. You went above and beyond in the way you cared for her, and to this day I believe you are the reason she is still alive.

It's hard to adequately sum up this convoluted journey in a few short pages. Writing every one of these sentences has been painful to remember, and I have not been able to do it without crying. These experiences we endured severely altered the person I am today. I made some misguided decisions along the way, but have also realized that the life I live will never be perfect. That is something I can accept. Not everything that was born from this struggle has been something I am ashamed of though.

I now realize all that Evelyn, my mother, has done and continues to do for me. She has always been the foundation of our family, helping us thrive to become the best person possible. She has sacrificed her mental health for her family, taking all of our problems into consideration and treating them with as much respect as she would treat her own. There were nights she mentioned she hadn't slept a single hour, due to the fact that she was instead praying for her family members to be healed. This was not something she was asked to do, but rather something she felt she needed to do.

In addition to constantly keeping her family's issues in mind, she also spearheaded the research into a possible medical diagnosis. She spent countless hours in front of our sluggishly slow computer, reading about medical conditions and contacting people who displayed some of the same effects as Teya. This dedication to the cause eventually paid off after five gruelling years, when her daughter was finally diagnosed with the correct illness. This psychological battle gave my mother a level of stress that is still unimaginable to me. It is hard enough for someone to truly take care of just themselves, but then to put the same level of work into each of your family member's poor health is mentally draining.

I can say without a doubt my mother cares for me. The sacrifices she made in order to keep all of us breathing for another day can only come from a place of authentic humbleness. This is a lesson I will always remember. Thank you Evelyn for showing me how to unconditionally love.

Seeing how immobilizing chronic pain can be I now have a new respect for Loni, my father, and the way he perseveres. I cannot remember a time when he did not have back, neck or headache related pain. The amount of stress his body and mind have endured is unbelievable, and the effects of this endurance are visible. Still that has never given him a reason to admit defeat. Everyday he gets up for work and refuses to let pain deprive him of living life. This reminds me that sometimes I let my small problems appear bigger than they actually are.

Applying the appropriate mindset to an issue can completely change your perspective. One time I asked my dad why he hadn't just given up on life yet? Nothing ever seemed to go right for him, yet he chose joy instead of anger. He responded by telling me "What if this is the best it ever gets?." This sentence has stuck with me since the day he said it, because it really rings true. So often we as a society are caught up on everything we don't have, instead of acknowledging the numerous things we do have.

Whenever I begin to feel like I'm in a bad situation, I think of my dad and his response. My dad is a man of few words, because the times he does speak he has something important to say. Thank you Loni for helping me view the glass as half full, and realizing the blessings I have instead of the ones I am lacking.

When I was introduced into the family my sister was upset. This little baby was receiving all the attention that she was so used to solely getting. Though as time went on the idea of being an older sibling started to sound appealing to her. She wanted to help her little brother who she felt was too naive to do anything. This loving relationship quickly flourished into something that was not just a phase. Growing up together we rarely fought or argued. Somehow we were opposites that paired together perfectly, and we could always depend on each other when we needed help.

When Teya's condition began to return with worsening intensities, I started avoiding her in an attempt to cope with the pain that I saw her enduring. For a pair that had been together since the beginning of time she was hurt by this, and she had a right to be offended. The way I left her to her own devices and pretended nothing was happening was vile and out of character for her sweet little brother. She began to feel lonely and betrayed that I seemed to no longer care for her. Our relationship did weaken because of this, however we both knew we still loved each other.

As much as hardships are tough when you're going through them, you often emerge from them stronger than when you started. That is exactly what happened to our family. We never stopped loving each other, it had just become more difficult to with all the obstacles blocking our path. These obstacles forced us to unite together as a group, as there was no way we could have beat the obstacles alone. I am now thankful for the terrible events that I have been through, even if I'm not proud of the path I took to get there. As a family I know that we have become more dependent on each other in a positive way. Poor health was, and still is, something our family struggles with, but it has never been able to completely prevent us from enjoying life.

While your pain did attack you like waves of mountains Teya, you never stopped climbing. You wanted to give up so many times but always pushed through hell, one period at a time. You refused to let the pain fully conquer your body and mind, even when all the odds seemed to be stacked against you. That is a strength that I don't know I would've been able to maintain for as long as you did.

I am truly sorry for the way I failed to support you. I am sorry that you had to go into the darkest part of your life without your brother by your side. Whether you knew it or not, watching you go through your transformation in the fierce form that you did was inspiring to me. Thank you Teya for showing me how to overcome, and never giving up on me.

Chapter 15: Describing My Endo Symptoms to a Medical Professional

Symptoms of Endometriosis:

- Chronic or intermittent pelvic pains
- Due to dysmenorrhea or neuropathy, endo can often cause back pain
- Spotting or bleeding between menstrual periods
- Menorrhagia- Heavy bleeding during menstrual cycle
- Painful menstruation, sex and orgasm
- Infertility - miscarriage or ectopic pregnancies
- Painful bowel movements, rectal pain
- Frequent urination, frequent yeast infections
- Bloating, gassiness, cramps, diarrhea or constipation
- Fatigue, aching, constant discomfort, nausea, headaches
- Contractions in the uterus
- General body weakness
- Irregular vaginal clotting
- Chemical sensitivities

I am a part of a number of very good Facebook Endo Support Groups. On a few of these sites I asked how endo girls try to describe their endo pain/symptoms to a medical professional. This is *not* a normal way of describing a "period." Endo cannot just be a bad period...there is an actual disease that gives incredible pain. This is how the Endo girls described it:

"It's like Freddy Kreuger is teaching an American Sign Language class in my abdomen."

"I feel like my insides want to be on my outside."

"The civil war, complete with cannons and bayonets, and my abdomen is the battlefield."

"I felt like an extra on Game of Thrones being run through with a sword."

"Evil leprechauns wearing sharpened soccer cleats tap dancing on my uterus."

"Like my insides just lost a fight to a cheese grater."

"Someone is digging into me with a spoon, because at least knives and forks have sharp edges."

"Endo: like wearing a corset made of barbed wire that's pulled tighter and tighter whilst ninja stars are randomly thrown your way. Adhesions: like all my organs are fused together like Pangea."

Chapter 16: Things Not To Say to a Struggling Endo Girl

Preface: These are all things I have personally heard or things that people have said to my face. I do not hold resentment for most of these, but some, I am still working through. When running them by one of my Endo friends, she broke down crying and said, "This is so accurate and I've had almost all of these said to me!" This is not something made up, this is something experienced. If you have said any of these things to someone with Endo or *possibly* with Endo, please be brave enough to go back and tell them you were wrong. All these thoughts pile on top of each other in a struggling girls mind and even having one removed makes them not feel so "insane."

1. **"It's all in your head"** - Not only is this hurtful but horrible. This form of judging hurts so deeply. All Endo girls ever hear is that they are crazy and that 'it's all in your head'. When someone *knows* they are severely hurting, then they *know*. No one else gets to judge as they cannot see into that person's body. It's an invisible disease that's on the inside so only that person knows and feels what's truly wrong with them.

2. **"Stop being dramatic, it doesn't hurt that much"** – *Wow*! And yes, people often say that! What woman wants to live a life "faking" to be in that much pain. Doctors have said that the pain girls feel from

endometriosis or adenomyosis is equivalent to being in labour. If it's not your own body, you *cannot* judge if "it doesn't hurt that much."

3. **"It's just period cramps"** - It is *not just period cramps*! My mom reports that she had regular periods with pain that was easily fixed with over the counter drugs like Midol. This is not possible for an Endo girl. Regular periods do have pain, but not debilitation that makes narcotics a necessity. It is abnormal for a teenage girl to be missing out on the things she loves.

    For example, my mom thought at first when I had such bad pain around my periods it was because I was being dramatic. But when she had to pick me up from a movie with a few friends that I was thrilled about, she realized 'if it was just period cramps she would not have left the movie she was excited to see. This is something more serious'. (Also see chapter 18 for clarification of the difference).

4. **"Get over it"** - Trust me, if this struggling girl could "get over" no one believing her and "get over" feeling like something is seriously wrong with her, and that she feels hopeless, she gladly would have. Depression grasps *every* single person at some point who deals with chronic pain. No one has the right to tell someone else to "get over it" because they do not know what goes on behind the scenes. They don't know how the doctors are telling this sixteen-year-old girl to just, "Go get pregnant because that will fix everything," or how the side effects of the many pills they are told to take, is affecting them.

5. **"Just take Advil/ Tylenol"** - *They already have*!!! Endo girls have tried *everything*! They are struggling to find pain relief and that is why self-harm is often attempted. Not only this, but doctors flag their files as being "Drug Seekers: Do not listen to this patient because they complain about pain to get prescription pills." We sometimes go to great lengths to try to get pain relief. For instance, another Endo girl gave me synthetic weed to try, and Oxycodone pills. We literally try to help each other out, because we understand how critical it is to live this way. I'm not saying that sharing prescription pills is good, but it is better than no pain relief

so that attempting suicide seems like the only option. (This is a legit scenario of one of my Endo friends).

6. **"I don't see anything wrong with you!"** - Just because you don't see it, doesn't mean it's not there...like a brain or like Jesus. There are many, many endo groups on Facebook that I follow. Girls try to express their pain by drawing pictures of a uterus tied up in barbed wire, with a little man on the inside drilling into the side, and another person in the ovary lighting a grenade that will go off.

    Under pictures like that, are thousands of comments (literally) of girls agreeing and saying things like, "Finally a picture that shows honestly what my pain feels like." It's easier for a doctor to help people instantly if they can physically see the problem (a broken arm, a skin condition, a piece of metal in your eye). They jump to the rescue. The many women who are suffering and trying to get help, are silenced or pushed aside by doctors because when the doctor doesn't *see* anything wrong, then there must be nothing wrong. Internal issues, not visible to the eye, take longer to diagnose but they are there.

7. **"Why is it always all about you?"** – Yes, it seems the world always revolves around that one sister, friend, family member etc. who controls whether plans will go through or be cancelled. The thought is, 'mom is always taking care of my sister and bringing her food in bed and when I ask her to bring me something she tells me that she is 'busy with my sister', or 'that I'm well and I can get it myself'. This is hard, but honestly, no Endo girl can make it through this journey alone. We need help even if we don't want to admit it. It is true, friends or parents with a servant heart are selfless. Sometimes that is the only factor that helps one not feel that the last straw is suicide.

8. **"Just PRAY more"** - Anyone who is at wits end always is seen last resort praying. While for some it is their first resort for comfort. Endo girls always get Bible verses in letters or cards and sometimes the Bible is the only thing that we read, crying tears onto the page and begging for God to take this thorn from our flesh.

If you tell someone they need to pray more, then look at yourself. You are not with them every single minute and you do not know just how much they pray. Don't ever let yourself be in the judging position because you do not know the motives, lives, and reasons that people do things. Instead of saying pray more, you pray more for them. Or you can encourage them by saying "I will pray for you a lot more now that I know your situation."

9. **"Just have hope"** – The thing that Endo girls bounce back and forth between, is whether to keep hope close or push it as far away as possible. If you tell someone struggling with chronic pain to 'just keep hope' they are literally alive in front of you because that's what they are doing. It is when a person feels truly hopeless that they decide it's time to leave this earth. Everyone just keeps saying the word hope and soon after months or years of pain and hearing people say it over and over again you just push it away. Don't bring someone to that point. If they are in front of you, it is purely because there is a bit of hope left in them. Instead, maybe say, "I'm so sorry you're going through this."

10. **"Don't worry you will be healed yet"** - *You do not know that*!!! Do not give someone false hope! This is something else that is incredibly frustrating to hear as you feel trapped in this circle of pain that seems to never end and doctors, family or friends are not helping a single bit. Endo girls just want to hear a shred of truth from someone. Instead say, "I don't know if you will ever be fully healed, but I am sticking with you and helping you along." The saying "Truth will set you free," applies everywhere including here.

11. **"Maybe this is happening because you're supposed to learn something from this"** - That could be the truth but it's really not helpful at all to hear. If you really think that you can see so many things they can learn from this, then just pray for them that they see those things as well; without you telling them.

12. **"Maybe this is happening because you deserve it or because its karma for the evil you've done"** - First of all, I don't believe in karma. Read the first three chapters of Job from the Bible. There are many reasons why bad things happen to good people or that bad things happen for no reason at all. Plus, I don't believe any person has the authority or knowledge to be able to judge a person based on what they have done. You don't know their reasons, motives or situation for why they do things. Secondly, the girl you just said that too is bed ridden most of the time and doesn't even have the opportunity to do "bad things." It's the "healthy/well" people that have many more chances and situations to do bad things...not the girl restricted to her bed.

13. **"God let this happen to you"** - God does not put disease upon a person, Satan does this. Yes there was the fall of Man when Adam and Eve gave into temptation. The reason disease/chronic pain happen (from a Biblical view) is either A. Because of sin in the world, or B. Because Satan causes it. But, it always has to go through God's hands before Satan can allow this. I am thankful that God always knows what's going on and that everything passes by Him before it comes to me. Then I know, that no matter how terrible it is to me, God only ever has my best interest in mind. Read the first three chapters of Job from the Bible.

14. **"You just want attention"** - Girls who want attention are still able to do life. These girls can not. They miss doing things with their friends and family that they badly wanted to do. Why would a girl 'fake' being sick to get attention if she would be missing the movie she talked about five months before it came out or stays in bed all day when her favourite TV show is on? This is how you know she's not just wanting attention; when it wrecks the favourite parts of her life.

15. **"Why would you self harm if you apparently hurt?"** - Do you know how Marilyn Monroe died? She had endometriosis and she was trying to escape the pain. She overdosed on pain-killers due to her pain. When you hurt as intensely as Endo girls or girls with a rare form of endometriosis called adenomyosis, the urge to be in *some kind of control* of the

pain is there. I only attempted cutting three times and the only reason was to be in control of my own pain. It is hard not knowing what is happening to you.

Self-harm is a form of letting someone see physically that something is wrong. Doctors and others seem to think that, "If I can't see it, and it doesn't show up on scans, then it's not there." But, whenever a person sees someone else with cut marks up their arms, they suddenly see that something is wrong and this person needs help. Sometimes, self-harm is just a way to show people that there is something more going on inside; that people aren't seeing. But sadly, when they see the self-harm, they instantly assume you have a mental disorder.

16. **"You deserve this"** - I haven't met a single Endo girl who has said, "Oh I wish ____ would have this disease." Every girl always says, "I wouldn't wish this on my worst enemy," and they say that because it is true. *No one* deserves this amount of pain. It does not just hurt around a girl's period or just in the uterus, it affects every part of the body. I honestly don't think there is an evil enough person in the world that I would wish this on.

17. **"Are you pregnant?"**- Most of the time Endo girls main struggle is pain and infertility. The thing they want most in the world is to be able to be pregnant. It's most women's hearts desire, the thing they crave. If you think an Endo girl may be pregnant *do not ask her*! Ask her mom or her friend. Endo girls struggle with looking pregnant due to bloating from all the inflammation and they can only wish that that baby bump was a baby bump and not just inflammation swelling up their insides.

Chapter 17: How You Can Help an Endo Girl (Written by Jason Friesen)

When I first met Teya, we had both started attending Steinbach Bible College and had several classes together. As we interacted within the school setting, one of the first things she told me was that she suffered from chronic pain. This was the first time I had exposure to endometriosis. Now I wasn't completely taken aback by this kind of suffering, my mom had her own share of physical battles and pain.

But as Teya started telling me more about her life and her journey with endometriosis, I was shocked at everything people had done and said to her because of it. So many of the stories I heard from her and her parents were about people who judged her because of her physical sickness. Rather than take her word for it that she was in constant and intense pain, people either didn't believe it or they belittled it. After all, we can't see it, you look healthy, so just get over yourself. As much as her pain had shaped her, I believe that a person is more than their circumstances, so I chose to look deeper and find the girl behind the pain. And I found her.

We started dating in December of 2015, a few weeks after she was re-diagnosed with endometriosis. Looking back, she confessed that she was terrified at the time that I would lose interest in her when I found out she was sick again. This confused me. I struggled to understand why a guy would leave her because of her sickness. I told her and her parents many times that sickness sounded like one of the worst reasons to leave someone, even in a dating relationship.

But then she told me that that had happened, not to her but to others with this chronic pain as well. So to all endo girls out there: I am sorry that boys can be so ignorant and hurtful. Please don't give up on it all, there are some of us out there who do try to be good men. I won't promise that we will always live up to our own standards, but we will keep trying.

And to all the men, please don't be one of these guys. If you are lazy or selfish, please be honest enough to say that you are and that you are too immature to help someone else. If you're not ready to date a girl who has pain, then maybe you shouldn't date at all. Dating is more than the girl and more than what she gives you.

At the same time, thank you to all the men who are standing by a girl with endo. On one end of the spectrum, I don't think we understand how much it means to our girlfriends/wives that we have stayed by them through it all. On the other end, I think that we under-think it. I have had Teya and her parents thank me for seeing through it and being so kind and thoughtful. But honestly, I don't see myself acting any other way even if she didn't have pain. The model I try to follow isn't called "How to help girls with endo." The model I try to follow is "How to be a godly and good boyfriend and husband." The pain is irrelevant at this point. Oh sure, the application might look a bit different day to day, but the principle behind it stays the same.

We dated for a year during our first and second years of college. Shortly before Christmas break of our second year, I proposed to her and we got engaged. During all this time, there were many ups and downs, good days and bad days, people who were kind and people who were not. Through all of it, I tried to be a good boyfriend and then a good fiancé. I did my best to live by Jesus' model of love and gentleness, compassion and self-sacrifice that He did so very well, and also to live by the guidelines for relationships that are found in the Bible. This was my model for interacting with Teya, and sometimes I lived up to it, and other times I most definitely did not. But in all of it, we had a wonderful dating relationship that I don't regret at all, and it led to a marriage that I cannot imagine being without.

Alright, now to the actual subject matter of this chapter. So how can you help an Endo girl?

In the three-and-a-bit years that I have known Teya, I have learned to recognize a few things. In college, we had a pain scale from 1 to 10, 1 being low pain, and 10 being extreme pain. This leads to tip #1.

TIP 1: KEEP ASKING HOW SHE IS DOING.

This may sound superficial. And it can be. People ask each other all the time, "How are you?" And we have our superficial answers for those superficial questions. But it depends who asks. If your best friend asks you how it's going, your answer could be very different than someone you don't interact with that much.

When we were dating, I would ask her several times a day, "How bad is your pain?" When you ask repeatedly, it shows that you have kept in mind that they are suffering, you haven't forgotten them. It shows that you care. Over time, I got pretty good at reading her body language and facial expressions, to the point that I would guess specific numbers on the pain scale. Here we run into tip #2.

TIP 2: ASK HOW TO HELP.

With asking how to help, you not only show that you care, but you act on it as well. Again, it may not seem like much, but it speaks volumes to the one you are doing it for. It will often be something simple. With these small acts of service, you are actually killing two birds with one stone. You are living out your care and commitment, and you are making their lives easier and more comfortable at the same time.

Warming up heating bags is one example of something simple you can do to help. For many girls with endometriosis, having a source of heat against their belly helps alleviate the pain a little bit. Rice bags are a simple portable solution for this. The problem then is that they only hold their heat for about 30-45 minutes. During college, I would often take a short break in the class to run to the nearest microwave and heat up the rice bag so that Teya could make it through the rest of the class. I know that Teya almost always carried one of these heat bags in her backpack, and I made it a habit for several years to carry one as well.

Getting snacks is another simple way of helping them out. Here again you are mainly doing the walking for them so that they don't have to agitate an already painful situation. Motion such as walking and even standing can easily make the pain worse. It's so simple, it may be easy to think, "That's such a small thing, why not do it yourself?" But if it's such a small thing, then it shouldn't be a big deal that they ask you to do it!

One more example would be to pick them up or drop them off so they don't have to walk or be outside in cold temperatures. Especially in the Manitoba prairies, where we live, it can get outrageously cold during the winters. I learned very quickly that cold temperatures make endometriosis pain much worse. To counter this, there were times when I would drive her the short distance from the dormitory building to the main college building.

Other times I would give her a ride on my way back to the dormitory so that she wouldn't have to walk if she didn't think she could travel the distance. These examples are by no means the only ones possible. There are many other small ways that you can help them out and show your commitment. However, the theme behind them all is the same: Doing what you can to be a good partner and to make their lives easier and more comfortable.

On a side note, they may feel bad asking you to do something as simple as filling their water bottle or getting a snack for them. Tell them that you are here to help them and make their lives easier. If I was in constant abdominal pain I would want to walk as little as possible, and I'm sure the same is true for them. However, it is possible that she may be too shy, proud, or embarrassed to ask for help with even the little things. This is where it is important to read the situation and just do things to help her out, even if she doesn't ask you to.

TIP 3: BE COMMITTED.

This tip probably sums up the other two and then some. I can't count the number of times I asked if there was anything else I could do in the middle of a bad pain attack and her first response was simply and immediately "Stay." I knew before we started dating that Teya dealt with endometriosis, and that it affected most of her life in many different ways. But when I started dating her, that didn't matter. In our relationship, we ended up getting married.

Now I know that's not the case with everyone, and if a guy dates a girl with endo and they aren't the right fit for each other, I'm not saying that they should stay together or get married anyway. But in your relationship, act in such a way so that if you do break up down the road, she will know that it is not because of her chronic pain. Don't necessarily be committed to the relationship, but rather, be committed to her as long as you are in the relationship.

When Teya would say "Stay" she didn't necessarily mean "keep dating me." She meant "even if something happens and we break up, I need you as a friend." Let's face it. Endo girls don't have many friends and above all else they need friends. It's hard going through any kind of pain, but going through it feeling alone is much worse, and sadly, there have been those who thought the best option was to put an end to it all. Sometimes a friend who is willing to stick by you is what they need to make it through those moments.

I don't regret dating someone with chronic pain. In fact, it has shaped me into a better man. I am more grateful for the things in life that I still take for granted at times. My colds and headaches aren't that miserable. I can hold a job, and that is something I had always assumed for myself. But with a different perspective, things like this take on a different value. Yes, there are still bad days, but there are many good days too. I am grateful for what I have learned from Teya and her battle with health, and I know that there are still many wonderful moments and lessons coming.

Chapter 18:
Endometriosis vs. Cramps

CRAMPS	ENDOMETRIOSIS
Person A has their period. She has some cramps and feels uncomfortable.	Person B has endometriosis. She has had three surgeries to manage her endometriosis and still hasn't found relief.
Person A takes some ibuprofen; she's feeling better now.	Person B's prescription medication aren't helping. She may need to go to the ER for pain relief.
Person A's cramps are located just below her belly button.	Person B's cramps are in her pelvis, legs, back and make it difficult for her to go to the bathroom.

CRAMPS	ENDOMETRIOSIS
Person A uses a heating pad for her cramps. It's quite helpful.	Person B uses a heating pad and leaves it on so long she burns herself.
Person A gets ready to leave the house and packs some basics.	Person B gets ready to leave the house and packs a portable heating pad, extra underwear, tampons, pads, three pain medications, and two prescriptions for nausea.
Person A's period ends, and she feels better.	Person B's period ends, and she's still in significant pain.

While having cramps can suck, excruciating cramps are not normal and can be a sign of endometriosis. If someone opens up to you about having endometriosis, don't say, "Everyone gets cramps, that's just part of having your period." Listen[2].

Chapter 19: Endometriosis - Two Types of Surgeries: Ablation vs. Excision

Ablation: is a procedure to remove the thin inner lining of the uterus (through burning). It's usually done to reduce heavy menstrual bleeding, and is thought to be a way to help women who struggle with endometriosis.

Excision: is a surgical procedure in which the surgeon removes growths, scar tissue, and endometriosis while saving the healthy lining and tissues. To ensure all endometriosis is removed, removing the surrounding tissue where endo was found helps to get all "grains" of it left so it can not multiply and become as bad as before.

Understanding the difference between excision and ablation through the dandelion metaphor:

The dandelion metaphor is comparing Endo to having a dandelion in your lawn that you need to get rid of. The options are:

1. Colouring the dandelion green so that it blends in with the grass (hormone therapy)
2. Mowing the lawn (ablation surgery)
3. Digging out the dandelion knowing some of the roots are still in place (excision surgery)
4. Digging the dandelion out and removing a foot around it to get all the roots and seeds out (aggressive/deep/wide excision.) When it comes to a Partial hysterectomy (uterus only), it does help relieve the pain but only the pain that's on or in the uterus muscle. It does not help the Endo pain anywhere else in the abdomen/pelvic cavity. Having a full Hysterectomy (uterus and ovaries removed), will relieve the pain that's on the ovaries and uterus but will not relieve the pain in the pelvis or on any other organs.

In the past, it was believed that by having a full hysterectomy, they were removing all the hormones that fed endometriosis; however, through research, it has been discovered that endometriosis grows its own hormones, which continue to feed endo. This pain is only stopped by wide or aggressive excision surgery on the organs or in the pelvis where endo is present.

Being told to try all the "band aid" options first:

I asked Dr. Andrew Cook a few questions regarding what the best option is when thinking about ablation or excision and even asked about the Canadian doctors saying that girls must go through all the "band aid" options (such as Visanne, Lupron, IUD etc.) before they consider giving them surgery.

He said in regards to trying "band aid" options,

"The symptoms of endometriosis can vary significantly and their severity. What we are really talking about is quality of life. If the patient has no quality of life then a more aggressive treatment is appropriate. If the symptoms of endometriosis in a given individual are minor, then a more conservative approach would be appropriate. In general, if the patient is doing well overall, other than a couple days a month and the pain isn't severe, then, a trial of oral contraceptive pills would be an appropriate consideration, as long as the patient does not have significant side effects with this treatment.

In my experience, many women with endometriosis have significant side effects with hormonal treatment. If this is the case, I think it is important to understand that women with endometriosis are sensitive and the side effects are real and rather consistent no matter what type of hormonal treatment and thus this is probably not a good fit for the patient in question. If the oral contraceptive pills are used either cyclically or continuously and result in significant improvement in quality of life, they can be an effective temporary treatment keeping in mind they do not rid the body of endometriosis but have stopped pain and suffering. For many women though, oral contraceptive pills do not provide a significant improvement in quality of life and thus an alternative treatment should be considered.

Other medical treatments available include progesterone oral contraceptive pills or bioidentical progesterone or even injectable or implantable hormones. Other options include such things as Danocrine and GnRH agonist for/with the recent addition of or Orlissa GnRH antagonist. These latter medications often have severe side effects that resulted in a decrease in quality of life. This is due to the pain that it's meant to help treat."[3]

I then specifically asked about his opinion on women taking Lupron. I had tried this drug, and have experienced its' lasting side effects.

His response is as follows:

"I believe it is important for women to be fully informed of all her treatment options along with the pros and cons of each treatment option. In my experience, there are usually better treatment options than Lupron, especially Depo-Lupron. If a woman, after being fully informed of all the potential side effects, wishes to try this treatment, then I would suggest that they use a short acting form of the GnRH agonist or antagonist, such as Synarel or Orilissa, so if severe side effects are experienced she can immediately stop the medications. The short acting form will be out of her body within a week as opposed to the months and months for Depo-Lupron. I would not personally take Depo-Lupron as the first form of GnRH agonists or antagonist. In my experience, in dealing with women with endometriosis, their experience with Depo-Lupron is uniformly, with rare exception, very traumatized."[4]

ENDOMETRIOSIS

★
Always remember to speak with your surgeon about what makes sense for you, your body, and your specific case.

two types of surgery

ABLATION	vs	EXCISION
LIKE SLASH-AND-BURN		LIKE A TROWEL

Burning or vaporizing endometriosis at the surface with a laser or heat gun, leaving roots and other scar tissue behind.

Can cause additional scarring and allow lesions to grow back, similar to how slash-and-burn can damage the land and only temporarily clear brush.

Physically cutting out endometriosis lesions at the root and not leaving the disease behind.

Can be performed with surgical tools, a laser used as a knife, and robotic-assisted methods.

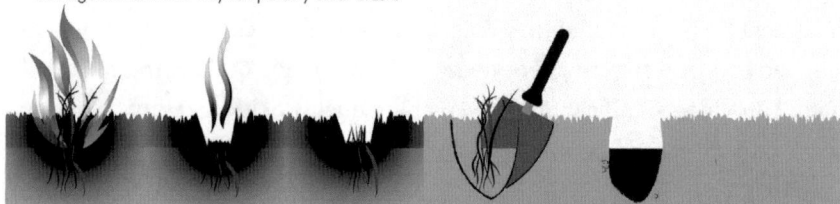

✓ PROS	✗ CONS	✓ PROS	✗ CONS
• Typically costs less, and is more likely to be covered by insurance	• High rates (40%-60%) of recurrence 1-2 years after surgery	• Long-term relief rates in skilled surgeons as high as 75%-85%	• Typically more expensive and less likely to be covered by insurance
• Shorter recovery time	• Underlying endometriosis and scar tissue not treated	• Ensures total removal of endometriosis detected by surgeon	• Even if 90% of disease is removed, complete remission not guaranteed
• Provides short-term relief	• Higher and earlier recurrence rates of endometriomas	• Allows for pathological diagnosis of tissue	• More invasive
• Less invasive	• Higher potential for complications & pain	• Significantly lower rates of endometrioma recurrence	• Less doctors specialize in excision
• More surgeons trained in ablation	• Higher risk of heat damaging underlying tissue or organs	• Higher precision means especially able to treat severe endometriosis	• Recovery can be longer
	• Burning means no specimens for pathological diagnosis		

Sources: The National Institute of Health, Endometriosis Australia, Center for Endometriosis Care

endographics.org
@endo_graphics

5

These options are the main options for removal of the disease. Doctors usually start by using "band aid" methods, sadly. While they do help control symptoms they do not fix the underlying problem. These help for quick relief but as soon as you stop you are back to square one if not worse. But finding a life of being pain free or very close comes from seeking out a surgery. This metaphor, originally by Sarah Sowers, shows clearly the pros and cons of both options.

While ablation is a less invasive surgery it is also less aggressive. Most women report that they were pain free about two to four years (in best cases) and then got all their pain and symptoms back. Excision, when performed aggressive enough; has given women many years pain free and if done by a skilled surgeon they reported never having those pains again.

When it comes to making a choice of which one is most reliable, Dr Cook encourages women that,

"There is no current medical treatment that has been proven to ensure appropriate rid of endometriosis. If conservative measures have been taken then surgery with wide excision of the endometriosis is appropriate. Surgery with coagulation, cautery or burning of the endometriosis is not appropriate, outdated and should be relegated to history books. Unfortunately this is still the most common type of surgery performed for endometriosis. The success rates are low and the recurrence rates are high, best explaining why so many women with endometriosis go through repetitive surgeries. In my practice most patients have undergone multiple surgeries before seeking my help and on average is the patient's fourth surgery for endometriosis but with the techniques that I use with (wide excision) the reoperation rate is 17 percent and endometriosis is seen in about half of these cases. Our outcome studying with up to fifteen-years of follow-up show 93 percent of women do not have recurrence of endometriosis and thus majority of women undergoing wide excision are actually cured of disease defined by endometrial implants in the pelvis."[6]

Chapter 20: Words from the Wise

To complete my interview with Dr. Cook who has helped many women under-stand their options and choices when it comes to endometriosis, a few other questions were asked and answered that I will put below. They are questions that I have wondered about personally, and maybe you have too and can gain some wisdom from these thorough answers. Enjoy!

What other diseases or conditions go with Endometriosis?

"This really raises the question of what actually endometriosis is. Is endome-triosis only endometrial implants in the pelvis or are there the implants just part of an overall disease process that involves many underlying problems with the patient's health?

If endometriosis was just a result of endometrial implants then wide excision surgery would be curative in the vast majority of patients of all her symptoms. We know that women with endometriosis often have numerous different co-morbidities associated with the endometrial implants including but not limited to autoimmune diseases, chronic fatigue, immune dysfunc-tion, multiple sensitivities including chemical sensitivities, food allergies, bowel and bladder symptoms including interstitial cystitis.

In my thirty-years of treating endo, about half of the patients I treat with wide excision surgery respond very well to surgery and are virtually 100 percent better. Other women have a whole list of conditions that result in ill health. Many years ago I coined the term Multiple System Dysfunction (MSD) to describe endometriosis patients that have a variety of issues that are not treated well with traditional Western medicine and most likely have at the core a whole range of underlying health issues ranging from genetic/epigenetic variations to environmental toxins, variations in the human microbiology and chronic intracellular infections to name a few.

At times some of these other conditions are mistaken for endometriosis and once lifestyle changes are implemented the symptoms that were thought to be a result of endometriosis resolve and in fact the patient never had endometriosis. I have said that endometriosis does not make a woman immune from experiencing any other health issues. It does seem that some patients have a degradation of the health that seems to be associated with endometriosis but certainly it is much more complex than just simply surgically removing all the diseased by wide excision. It is extremely important in these situations that a variety of different approaches are used to help and wellness be instituted and that a comprehensive enough plan is put in place to make forward progress and regaining health."[7]

Can women be born with Endo?

"It is becoming more evident that endometriosis is probably a congenital condition rather than an acquired disease and thus by definition is the result of it being present at birth. It is not activated until puberty with the onset of estrogen production. At this time, we do not completely understand the exact pathophysiology or mechanism by which endometriosis forms."[8]

Why does having a baby not fix everything?

(I asked this, as this was what one doctor was recommending I do to "fix" my uterus problems).

"I think the real question is why would having the baby fix everything? We do know that there are immune changes that occur during pregnancy and that a woman does not have periods for about a year. The idea that endometriosis will be cured by pregnancy is a myth."[9]

Endnotes

1   Dr. Andrew Cook, MD, FACOG
2   "Chronic Illness on The Mighty." Facebook - Log In or Sign Up, 1 Mar. 2017, www.facebook.com/ChronicIllnessOnThemighty/.
3   Dr. Andrew Cook, MD, FACOG
4   Dr. Andrew Cook, MD, FACOG
5   "Home Page." Endographics.org, Sarah Digby, Sept. 2018, www.endographics.org/infographics/surgeries.
6   Dr. Andrew Cook, MD, FACOG
7   Dr. Andrew Cook, MD, FACOG
8   Dr. Andrew Cook, MD, FACOG
9   Dr. Andrew Cook, MD, FACOG

Printed in Canada